S0-CWY-111

The Complete Ninja Foodi Cookbook 2019

Easy, Healthy and Fast Ninja Foodi Pressure Cooker Recipes That Anyone Can Cook

By Judy Stella

Copyright ©2019 By Judy Stella
All rights reserved.

No part of this guide may be reproduced in any form without permission in writing from the publisher except in the case of brief quotations embodied in critical articles or reviews.

Legal & Disclaimer

The information contained in this book and its contents is not designed to replace or take the place of any form of medical or professional advice; and is not meant to replace the need for independent medical, financial, legal or other professional advice or services, as may be required. The content and information in this book has been provided for educational and entertainment purposes only.

The content and information contained in this book has been compiled from sources deemed reliable, and it is accurate to the best of the Author's knowledge, information and belief. However, the Author cannot guarantee its accuracy and validity and cannot be held liable for any errors and/or omissions. Further, changes are periodically made to this book as and when needed. Where appropriate and/or necessary, you must consult a professional (including but not limited to your doctor, attorney, financial advisor or such other professional advisor) before using any of the suggested remedies, techniques, or information in this book.

Upon using the contents and information contained in this book, you agree to hold harmless the Author from and against any damages, costs, and expenses, including any legal fees potentially resulting from the application of any of the information provided by this book. This disclaimer applies to any loss, damages or injury caused by the use and application, whether directly or indirectly, of any advice or information presented, whether for breach of contract, tort, negligence, personal injury, criminal intent, or under any other cause of action.

Table of Content

Delicious Breakfast Recipes

Morning Hashes

Preparation time: 5 minutes
Cooking time: 20 minutes
Total time: 25 minutes
Servings: 2

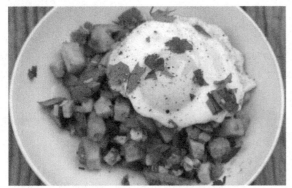

Ingredients:

- One tablespoon unsalted butter
- ½ teaspoon dried thyme, crushed
- ½ cup cauliflower florets, boiled and chopped
- ½ small onion, chopped
- ½ cup of water
- Salt and black pepper, to taste
- ½ pound turkey meat, chopped
- ¼ cup heavy cream

How to prepare:

1. Turn on the Ninja Foodi and press sauté.
2. Add butter and onions and sauté for 3 minutes.
3. Add cauliflowers and sauté for 2 minutes.
4. Add turkey and water.
5. Close the lid.
6. Set the Ninja Foodi to "Manual" at high pressure for 10 minutes, release the pressure quickly.
7. Open the lid and press broil.
8. Add heavy cream, cook for 2 minutes.
9. Serve and enjoy.

Nutritional Values:

Calories 151 , Total Fat 11.6 g , Saturated Fat 4.6 g , Cholesterol 335 mg , Sodium 144 mg , Total Carbs 0.7 g , Fiber 0 g , Sugar 0.7 g , Protein 11.1 g

Scrambled Cheese Eggs with Broccoli

Preparation time: 10 minutes
Cooking time: 8 minutes
Total time: 18 minutes
Servings: 6

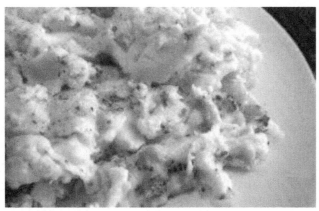

Ingredients:

- 2 tablespoons butter
- 12 ounces broccoli florets
- Salt and black pepper, to taste
- ¼ cup of water
- ¾ cup cheddar cheese, shredded
- 8 eggs
- 2 tablespoons milk

How to prepare:

1. Turn on Ninja Foodi and select sauté.
2. Add in butter, broccoli and sauté for 3 minutes.
3. Add in water, pepper, and salt and close the lid.
4. Set the Ninja Foodi to "Manual" at high pressure for 7 minutes, release the pressure quickly.
5. Open the lid and select sauté.
6. Add in eggs, milk and sauté for 2 minutes.
7. Add cheese and press "air crisp" at 320 degrees F.
8. Cook for 2 minutes and serve.

Nutritional Values:

Calories 197 , Total Fat 14.6 g , Saturated Fat 7.3 g , Cholesterol 244 mg , Sodium 219 mg , Total Carbs 4.7 g , Fiber 1.5 g , Sugar 1.7 g , Protein 12.7 g

Spinach Quiche

Preparation time: 15 minutes
Cooking time: 33 minutes
Total time: 48 minutes
Servings: 06

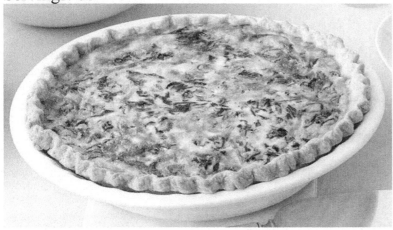

Ingredients:

- 1 tablespoon butter, melted
- 1 (10-ounce) package frozen spinach, thawed
- 5 organic eggs, beaten
- Salt and black pepper, to taste
- 3 cups Monterey Jack cheese, shredded

How to prepare:

1. Turn on Ninja Foodi and select sauté.
2. Add butter, spinach and sauté for 3 minutes.
3. Dish it out in a bowl.
4. Add in eggs, cheese, salt, pepper to a bowl.
5. Transfer it into molds which were greased.
6. Place molds inside Ninja Foodi and press "bake/roast."
7. Set the timer to 30 minutes at 360 degrees F and press start.
8. Remove molds after the time and cut in equal sized wedges.
9. Serve and enjoy.

Nutritional Values:

Calories 349 , Total Fat 27.8 g , Saturated Fat 14.8 g , Cholesterol 229 mg , Sodium 532 mg , Total Carbs 3.2 g , Fiber 1.3 g , Sugar 1.3 g , Protein 23 g

Mushroom Tofu

Preparation time: 15 minutes
Cooking time: 10 minutes
Total time: 25 minutes
Servings: 6

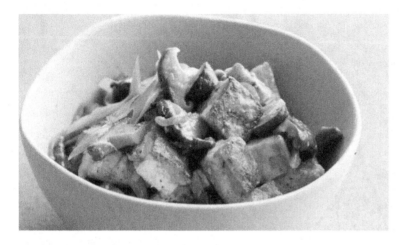

Ingredients:

- 8 tablespoons Parmesan cheese, shredded
- 2 cups fresh mushrooms, finely chopped
- 2 blocks tofu, pressed and cubed into 1-inch pieces
- Salt and black pepper, to taste
- 8 tablespoons butter

How to prepare:

1. Take a bowl and add tofu, salt, pepper in it. Mix well.
2. Press sauté and add in butter, tofu in a bowl and sauté for 5 minutes.
3. Add in mushrooms, parmesan cheese and sauté for 3 minutes.
4. Press air crisp and cool for 2 minutes at 350 degrees F.
5. Serve and enjoy.

Nutritional Values:

Calories 211 , Total Fat 18.5 g , Saturated Fat 11.5 g , Cholesterol 51 mg , Sodium 346 mg , Total Carbs 2 g , Fiber 0.4 g , Sugar 0.5 g , Protein 11.5 g

Bacon and Veggies

Preparation time: 10 minutes
Cooking time: 25 minutes
Total time: 35 minutes
Servings: 4

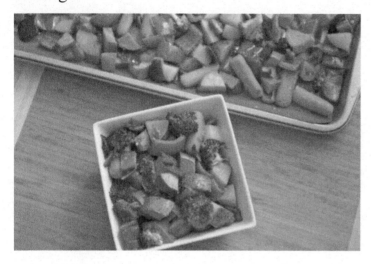

Ingredients:
- 1 green bell pepper, seeded and chopped
- 4 bacon slices
- ½ cup Parmesan Cheese
- 1 tablespoon avocado mayonnaise
- 2 scallions, chopped

How to prepare:
1. Place bacon at the bottom of Ninja Foodi.
2. Top it with avocado, mayonnaise, scallions, bell peppers, and parmesan cheese.
3. Press "bake/roast" and set the timer to 25 minutes at 365 degrees F.
4. Dish out and serve.

Nutritional Values:
Calories 197 , Total Fat 13.8 g , Saturated Fat 5.8 g , Cholesterol 37 mg , Sodium 662 mg , Total Carbs 4.7 g , Fiber 0.6 g , Sugar 1.9 g , Protein 14.3 g

Scrambled Onion Tofu

Preparation time: 10 minutes
Cooking time: 12 minutes
Total time: 22 minutes
Servings: 4

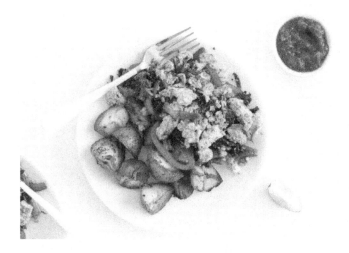

Ingredients:
- 4 tablespoons butter
- 2 blocks tofu, pressed and cubed into 1-inch pieces
- Salt and black pepper, to taste
- 1 cup cheddar cheese, grated
- 2 medium onions, sliced

How to prepare:
1. Take a bowl and add tofu, salt, pepper in it. Mix well.
2. Turn on the Ninja Foodi and select sauté.
3. Add in onions, butter and sauté for 3 minutes.
4. Add in tofu and cook for 2 minutes.
5. Add cheddar cheese and lock the lid.
6. Set Ninja Foodi on "air crisp" to 3 minutes at 340 degrees F.
7. Serve and enjoy.

Nutritional Values:
Calories 184 , Total Fat 12.7 g , Saturated Fat 7.3 g , Cholesterol 35 mg , Sodium 222 mg , Total Carbs 6.3 g , Fiber 1.6 g , Sugar 2.7 g , Protein 12.2 g

Omelet with Pepperoni

Preparation time: 10 minutes
Cooking time: 30 minutes
Total time: 40 minutes
Servings: 4

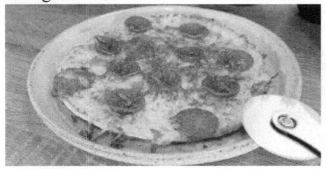

Ingredients:

- 4 tablespoons heavy cream
- 15 pepperoni slices
- 2 tablespoons butter
- Salt and black pepper, to taste
- 6 eggs

How to prepare:

1. Take a bowl and add eggs, heavy cream, salt, pepper, pepperoni and mix well.
2. Turn on the Ninja Foodi and select sauté.
3. Add in butter, egg mixture and sauté for 3 minutes.
4. Flip the side and lock the lid.
5. Set it on "air crisp" and cook for 2 minutes at 350 degrees F.
6. Serve and enjoy.

Nutritional Values:

Calories 141 , Total Fat 11.3 g , Saturated Fat 3.8 g , Cholesterol 181 mg , Sodium 334 mg , Total Carbs 0.6 g , Fiber 0 g , Sugar 0.5 g , Protein 8.9 g

Egg Bake with Ham & Spinach

Preparation time: 10 minutes
Cooking time: 30 minutes
Total time: 40 minutes
Servings: 8

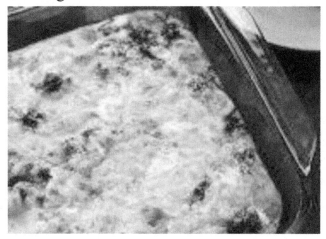

Ingredients:

- 3 pounds fresh baby spinach
- 6 eggs
- ½ cup cream
- 28-ounces ham, sliced
- 4 tablespoons butter, melted
- Salt and freshly ground black pepper, to taste

How to prepare:

1. Turn on the Ninja Foodi and select sauté.
2. Add in butter, spinach and sauté for 3 minutes.
3. Add in cream, ham slices, salt, pepper on top and close the lid.
4. Set it to "bake/roast" for 8 minutes at 360 degrees f.
5. Dish out and serve.

Nutritional Values:

Calories 188 , Total Fat 12.4 g , Saturated Fat 4.4 g , Cholesterol 53 mg , Sodium 1098 mg , Total Carbs 4.9 g , Fiber 2 g , Sugar 0.3 g , Protein 14.6 g

Scrambled Sausage with Cheese

Preparation time: 10 minutes
Cooking time: minutes
Total time: minutes
Servings: 4

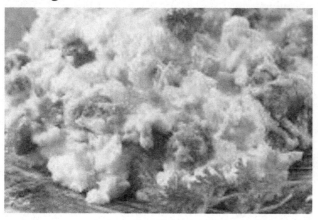

Ingredients:

- 4 eggs
- 4 cooked sausages, sliced
- 2 tablespoons butter
- ½ cup mozzarella cheese, grated
- ½ cup cream

How to prepare:

1. Take a bowl and add eggs, cream and mix well.
2. Pour this mixture in the Ninja Foodi.
3. Top it evenly with cheese and sausage slices.
4. Press "bake/roast" and set the timer to 20 minutes at 345 degrees F.
5. Dish out and serve.

Nutritional Values:

Calories 307 , Total Fat 25 g , Saturated Fat 5 g , Cholesterol 16 mg , Sodium 372 mg , Total Carbs 16 g , Fiber 5 g , Sugar 4 g , Protein 10 g

Bok Choy Samba with Bacon

Preparation time: 10 minutes
Cooking time: 14 minutes
Total time: 24 minutes
Servings: 06

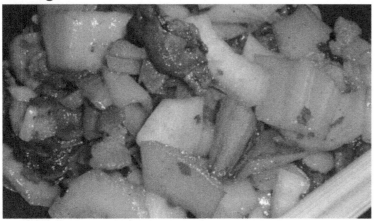

Ingredients:

- 4 bacon slices
- 2 tablespoons olive oil
- 8 tablespoons cream
- 8 bok choy, sliced
- 1 cup Parmesan cheese, grated
- Salt and black pepper, to taste

How to prepare:

1. Season the bok choy with salt and pepper.
2. Turn on Ninja Foodi and select sauté.
3. Add olive oil, bacon slices and sauté for 5 minutes.
4. Add in cream, seasoned bok choy and sauté for 6 minutes.
5. Top with parmesan cheese and lock the lid.
6. Set it on "air crisp" for 3 minutes at 350 degrees at F.
7. Dish out and enjoy.

Nutritional Values:

Calories 112 , Total Fat 4.9 g , Saturated Fat 1.9 g , Cholesterol 10 mg , Sodium 355 mg , Total Carbs 1.9 g , Fiber 0.4 g , Sugar 0.8 g , Protein 3 g

Healthy Vegetarian & Vegan Recipes

Spinach with Cheese

Preparation time: 10 minutes
Cooking time: 15 minutes
Total time: 25 minutes
Servings: 6

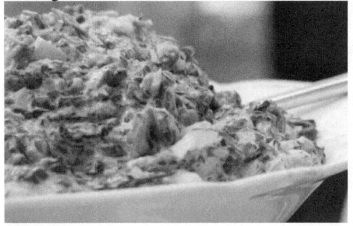

Ingredients:

- 4 tablespoons butter
- 2 pounds spinach, chopped and boiled
- Salt and black pepper, to taste
- 2/3 cup Kalamata olives, halved and pitted
- 1½ cups feta cheese, grated
- 4 teaspoons fresh lemon zest, grated

How to prepare:

1. Take a bowl and mix spinach, butter, salt, pepper in it.
2. Place the basket in Ninja Foodi and add spinach on it.
3. Select "air crisp" and set the timer to 15 minutes at 340 degrees F.
4. Dish out and serve.

Nutritional Values:

Calories 247 , Total Fat 18.7 g , Saturated Fat 3.3 g , Cholesterol 5 mg , Sodium 335 mg , Total Carbs 7.2 g , Fiber 3.9 g , Sugar 2.3 g , Protein 9.9 g

Veggies in Cheese

Preparation time: 10 minutes
Cooking time: 30 minutes
Total time: 40 minutes
Servings: 6

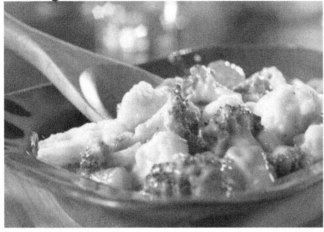

Ingredients:

- 2 onions, sliced thinly
- 2 tomatoes, sliced thinly
- 2 zucchini, sliced
- 2 teaspoons olive oil
- 2 cups cheddar cheese, grated
- 2 teaspoons mixed dried herbs
- Salt and freshly ground black pepper, to taste

How to prepare:

1. Add all ingredients in the Ninja Foodi and close the lid.
2. Select "air crisp" with time 3o minutes at 350 degrees F.
3. Open the lid, serve and enjoy.

Nutritional Values:

Calories 305 , Total Fat 22.3 g , Saturated Fat 13.2 g , Cholesterol 64 mg , Sodium 370 mg , Total Carbs 8.3 g , Fiber 2.9 g , Sugar 4.2 g , Protein 15.2 g

Broccoli Florets

Preparation time: 5 minutes
Cooking time: 6 minutes
Total time: 11 minutes
Servings: 6

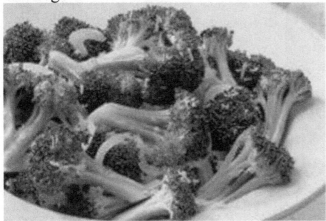

Ingredients:

- 4 tablespoons butter, melted
- Salt and black pepper, to taste
- 2 pounds broccoli florets
- 1 cup whipping cream

How to prepare:

1. Place the basket in the Ninja Foodi and add water.
2. Place florets on the basket and close the lid.
3. Select "pressure" with a timer 4 minutes and quickly release the pressure.
4. Open the lid, place florets in pot and season with salt and pepper.
5. Select "air crisp" and cook for 3 minutes at 360 degrees F.
6. Dish out and serve.

Nutritional Values:

Calories 178 , Total Fat 14.4 g , Saturated Fat 8.7 g , Cholesterol 43 mg , Sodium 111 mg , Total Carbs 9.6 g , Fiber 3.9 g , Sugar 2.6 g , Protein 4.7 g

Cauliflower Mash

Preparation time: 15 minutes
Cooking time: 5 minutes
Total time: 20 minutes
Servings: 6

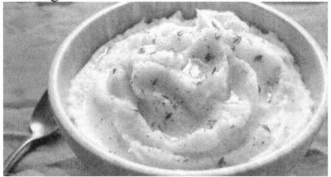

Ingredients:

- 1 tablespoon butter, softened
- ½ cup feta cheese
- Salt and black pepper, to taste
- 1 large head cauliflower, chop into large pieces
- 1 garlic clove, minced
- 2 teaspoons fresh chives, minced

How to prepare:

1. Place the basket in the bottom of the Ninja Foodi and add water.
2. Place cauliflower on the basket and lock the lid.
3. Select "pressure" with a timer for 5 minutes and do a quick release.
4. Open the lid and dish it out in a bowl.
5. Transfer it in an immersion blender and add all ingredients.
6. Blend till desired consistency has reached.
7. Serve and enjoy.

Nutritional Values:

Calories 124 , Total Fat 9.3 g , Saturated Fat 6.2 g , Cholesterol 32 mg , Sodium 333 mg , Total Carbs 6.1 g , Fiber 2.3 g , Sugar 3.2 g , Protein 5.4 g

Brussels Sprouts

Preparation time: 5 minutes
Cooking time: 6 minutes
Total time: 11 minutes
Servings: 8

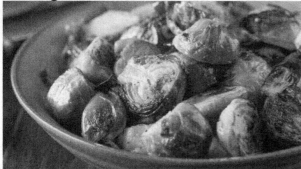

Ingredients:

- 2 pounds Brussels sprouts, trimmed and halved
- 1 cup almonds, chopped
- 1 tablespoon unsalted butter, melted

How to prepare:

1. Place the basket in the bottom of the Ninja Foodi and add water.
2. Place Brussel sprouts on the basket and lock the lid.
3. Select "pressure" with a timer for 3 minutes and do a quick release.
4. Open the lid and dish it out in a bowl.
5. Transfer Brussels sprouts and all other ingredients into the pot.
6. Select "air crisp" for 3 minutes at 350 degrees F.
7. Serve and enjoy.

Nutritional Values:

Calories 130 , Total Fat 7.8 g , Saturated Fat 1.5 g , Cholesterol 39 mg , Sodium 39 mg , Total Carbs 8.9 g , Fiber 5.7 g , Sugar 3 g , Protein 6.4 g

Green Beans

Preparation time: 5 minutes
Cooking time: 5 minutes
Total time: 10 minutes
Servings: 4

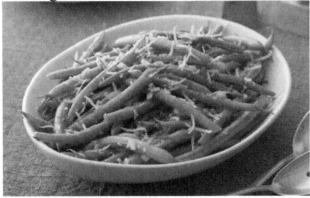

Ingredients:

- 1 pound fresh green beans
- 2 tablespoons butter
- 1 garlic clove, minced
- Salt and freshly ground black pepper, to taste
- 1½ cups water

How to prepare:

1. Add all ingredients in the Ninja Foodi and close the lid.
2. Select "pressure" and cook for 5 minutes, do a quick release.
3. Open the lid, dish out and serve.

Nutritional Values:

Calories 87 , Total Fat 5.9 g , Saturated Fat 3.7 g , Cholesterol 91 mg , Sodium 96 mg , Total Carbs 8.4 g , Fiber 3.9 g , Sugar 1.6 g , Protein 2.2 g

Vegetable Casserole

Preparation time: 15 minutes
Cooking time: 9 minutes
Total time: 24 minutes
Servings: 8

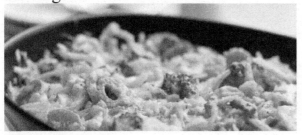

Ingredients:

- ½ cup almond flour
- Salt and black pepper, to taste
- 1 medium zucchini, chopped
- 1½ cups mozzarella cheese, shredded
- ½ cup unsweetened almond milk
- 8 large organic eggs
- 1 cup tomato, chopped
- 1 medium green bell pepper, seeded and chopped

How to prepare:

1. Place trivet at the bottom of Ninja Foodi and add water.
2. Take a bowl and mix in milk, flour, eggs, salt, and pepper.
3. Add in vegetables, cheese and mix well.
4. Add this mixture in baking dish and baking dish on trivet.
5. Close the lid and select "pressure."
6. Set the timer to 30 minutes with a natural release.
7. Open the lid and serve.

Nutritional Values:

Calories 102 , Total Fat 9.6 g , Saturated Fat 2.4 g , Cholesterol 61 mg , Sodium 139 mg , Total Carbs 5.1 g , Fiber 1.6 g , Sugar 2.2 g , Protein 10 g

Cauliflower Cheese

Preparation time: 10 minutes
Cooking time: 30 minutes
Total time: 40 minutes
Servings: 5

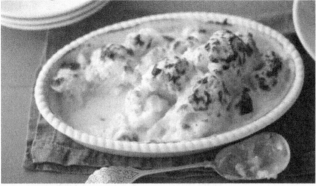

Ingredients:

- 1 tablespoon prepared mustard
- 1 head cauliflower
- 1 teaspoon avocado mayonnaise
- ½ cup Parmesan cheese, grated
- ¼ cup butter, cut into small pieces

How to prepare:

1. Add butter, cauliflower in Ninja Foodi and select sauté.
2. Sauté for 3 minutes.
3. Add in remaining ingredients and close the lid.
4. Select "pressure" and timer to 30 minutes with a natural release.
5. Open the lid and serve.

Nutritional Values:

Calories 155 , Total Fat 13.3 g , Saturated Fat 8.3 g , Cholesterol 37 mg , Sodium 280 mg , Total Carbs 3.8 g , Fiber 1.4 g , Sugar 1.4 g , Protein 6.7 g

Carrot and Zucchini

Preparation time: 10 minutes
Cooking time: 35 minutes
Total time: 45 minutes
Servings: 6

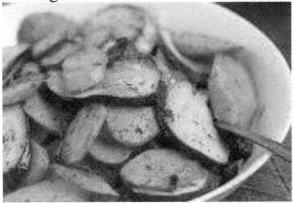

Ingredients:

- 6 teaspoons butter, divided and melted
- 2 pounds zucchini, sliced
- ½ pound carrots, sliced and peeled
- 1 tablespoon basil, chopped
- Salt to taste
- Black pepper to taste

How to prepare:

1. Add all ingredients and close the lid.
2. Select "pressure" and timer to 35 minutes with a natural release.
3. Open the lid and serve.

Nutritional Values:

Calories 74 , Total Fat 4.1 g , Saturated Fat 2.5 g , Cholesterol 10 mg , Sodium 95 mg , Total Carbs 8.8 g , Fiber 2.6 g , Sugar 4.5 g , Protein 2.2 g

Garlic Broccoli

Preparation time: 10 minutes
Cooking time: 12 minutes
Total time: 22 minutes
Servings: 8

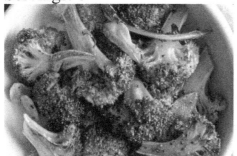

Ingredients:

- 2 tablespoons butter
- 8 garlic cloves, crushed
- 6 cups broccoli florets
- ½ cup parmesan cheese, grated
- 3 cups of water
- 1/8 teaspoon red pepper flakes, crushed
- Salt to taste

How to prepare:

1. Place all ingredients in the ninja pot and select sauté.
2. Sauté for 5 minutes and place florets in a plate.
3. Place basket in the Ninja Foodi.
4. Place florets on the basket and close the lid.
5. Select "pressure" with a timer 4 minutes and quickly release the pressure.
6. Open the lid, place florets in pot and season with salt and pepper.
7. Select "air crisp" and cook for 3 minutes at 360 degrees F.

 Dish out and serve.

Nutritional Values:

Calories 59 , Total Fat 3.5 g , Saturated Fat 2.1 g , Cholesterol 9 mg , Sodium 82 mg , Total Carbs 5.6 g , Fiber 1.8 g , Sugar 1.2 g , Protein 2.7 g

Pasta Recipes

Mac n Cheese

Preparation time: 15 minutes
Cooking time: 31 minutes
Total time: 46 minutes
Servings: 6

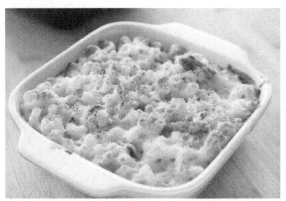

Ingredients:

- 1 can butternut squash puree
- 12 ounce frozen cauliflower rice
- 5 cups water, divided
- 1 cup heavy cream
- 16-ounce dry cavatappi pasta
- 1 teaspoon kosher salt
- 2 cups cheddar cheese, grated
- 6 ounce cream cheese
- Black pepper to taste
- ¼ cup unsalted butter, melted
- ¾ cup panko bread crumbs
- ½ cup shredded parmesan cheese
- 1 tablespoon fresh parsley, minced

How to prepare:

1. Add all ingredients in the Ninja Foodi except cheese and 1 cup water.
2. Close the lid and select "pressure."
3. Set the timer to 2 minutes at "high."
4. Do a natural release for 10 minutes and then a quick release.
5. Open the lid and add remaining ingredients.
6. Close the lid and select "broil."
7. Set timer to 9 minutes.

8. Open the lid mix well and serve instantly.

Nutritional Values:

Calories 1314 , Total Fat 80.9 g , Saturated Fat 40.1 g , Cholesterol 330 mg , Sodium 1849 mg , Total Carbs 64.6 g , Fiber 12.8 g , Sugar 11.2 g , Protein 76.8 g

Pasta Fagioli

Preparation time: 10 minutes
Cooking time: 14 minutes
Total time: 24 minutes
Servings: 8

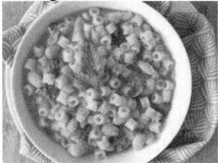

Ingredients:

- 1 tablespoon olive oil
- ½ tablespoon spicy Italian sausage, crumbled
- 1 onion, peeled and chopped
- ½ cup carrot, peeled and diced
- ½ cup celery, diced
- 2 cloves garlic, minced
- ½ teaspoon kosher salt
- ¼ teaspoon pepper
- 2 sprigs fresh rosemary
- 2 sprigs fresh thyme
- 2 cans great northern beans, drained and rinsed
- 2 cups tomatoes, crushed
- 6 cups chicken stock
- 1½ cups pasta

How to prepare:

1. Turn on the Ninja Foodi and select sauté let it heat for 5 minutes.
2. Add oil, sausage and cook till sausage is cooked.
3. Add in remaining ingredients and cook for 5 minutes, stirring continuously.
4. Close the lid and select "pressure."
5. Set timer to 4 minutes at "high," do a quick release.
6. Open the lid and serve.

Nutritional Values:

Calories 357 , Total Fat 3.5 g , Saturated Fat 0.8 g , Cholesterol 0 mg , Sodium 747 mg , Total Carbs 62.9 g , Fiber 20.2 g , Sugar 4.8 g , Protein 21.4 g

Pepperoni Pizza Pasta

Preparation time: 15 minutes
Cooking time: 30 minutes
Total time: 45 minutes
Servings: 8

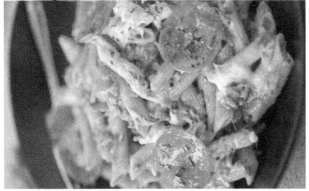

Ingredients:

- 1 onion, peeled and cut in half
- 2tablespoons extra virgin olive oil
- 1 teaspoon kosher salt
- ½ teaspoon dried oregano
- ½ teaspoon dried basil
- ¼ teaspoon ground black pepper
- ¼ teaspoon crushed red pepper
- 6 cloves garlic, minced
- 1 can tomatoes
- 1 can tomato puree
- 1 cup red wine
- 2 cups chicken stock, divided
- 1 pepperoni sausage, cut in small pieces
- 16 ounces dry rigatoni pasta
- 4 cups mozzarella cheese, shredded and divided
- 1 package pepperoni, thinly sliced

How to prepare:

1. Turn on the Ninja Foodi and select sauté let it heat for 5 minutes.
2. Add in oil, onions and cook for 2 minutes.
3. Add in remaining ingredients except cheese and pepperoni slices stir continuously.
4. Close the lid and select "pressure."
5. Set the timer to 6 minutes at "high."
6. Do a natural release for 10 minutes and then a quick release.

7. Open the lid and add cheese, topped with pepperoni slices.
8. Close the lid and select "air crisp" with a timer for 5 minutes at 400 degrees F.
9. Open the lid and serve.

Nutritional Values:

Calories 560 , Total Fat 20.4 g , Saturated Fat 7 g , Cholesterol 73 mg , Sodium 1141 mg , Total Carbs 67.6 g , Fiber 2.9 g , Sugar 6.6 g , Protein 23.4 g

Penne and Sausage Ragu

Preparation time: 15 minutes
Cooking time: 18 minutes
Total time: 33minutes
Servings: 6

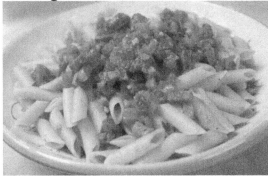

Ingredients:

- 2 tablespoons canola oil
- 1 lb Italian sausages, casings removed
- 1 lb smoked sausage, diced
- 2 carrots, peeled and diced
- 4 stalks celery, diced
- 1 onion, diced
- 4 garlic cloves, minced
- 48 ounce roasted red peppers, strained and pureed
- 1 cup chicken stock
- 1 cup heavy cream
- 1 tablespoon kosher salt
- 1 tablespoon fresh rosemary, minced
- 1 box dry penne pasta
- 1 cup mozzarella cheese, shredded

How to prepare:

1. Turn on the Ninja Foodi and select sauté.
2. Let it heat for 5 minutes.
3. Add in oil, sausages and cook for 5 minutes, stirring and breaking the meat.
4. Add in carrots, celery, onion, garlic and cook for 5 minutes.
5. Add in remaining ingredients except for mozzarella and stir well.
6. Close the lid and select "pressure."
7. Set the timer to 3 minutes at "low."
8. Do a quick release and then open the lid.
9. Mix well and add in mozzarella.
10. Close lid, select "broil" with a timer to 5 minutes.

11. Open the lid and serve.

Nutritional Values:

Calories 1462 , Total Fat 64.6 g , Saturated Fat 21.8 g , Cholesterol 338 mg , Sodium 3076 mg , Total Carbs 160.4 g , Fiber 4.1 g , Sugar 12.1 g , Protein 59 g

Meatballs Pasta Bake

Preparation time: 15 minutes
Cooking time: 30 minutes
Total time: 45 minutes
Servings: 10

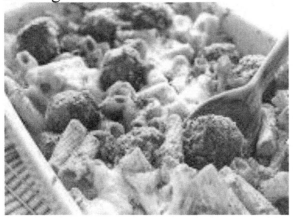

Ingredients:

- 2 lbs ground beef, uncooked
- 2 large eggs
- ½ cup parmesan cheese, grated
- ¼ cup milk
- ½ cup seasoned bread crumbs
- ½ cup parsley, chopped
- 2 teaspoons granulated garlic
- 2 teaspoons kosher salt
- 3 tablespoons olive oil
- 48-ounce marinara sauce
- 1 cup of water
- 1 cup dry red wine
- 1 box dry cavatappi pasta
- 1 cup ricotta cheese
- 1 cup mozzarella cheese, shredded

How to prepare:

1. Take a bowl and add beef, eggs, cheese, milk, crumbs, parsley, garlic and salt in it.
2. Mix well till combined.
3. Form 20 meatballs and set aside.
4. Turn on Ninja Foodi and select sauté and heat it for 5 minutes.
5. Add in oil and meatballs, when they are browned, transfer them in a bowl.
6. Add in marinara sauce, water, wine, pasta in the pot and stir well.

7. Close the lid and select "pressure."
8. Set the timer to 2 minutes at "low."
9. Do a natural release for 10 minutes and then a quick release.
10. Open the lid and select sauté.
11. Add in meatballs, mix and simmer for 10 minutes.
12. Stir in all the cheese and close the lid.
13. Select "bake/roast" for 5 minutes at 325 degrees F.
14. Open the lid and serve.

Nutritional Values:

Calories 431 , Total Fat 17.7 g , Saturated Fat 5.9 g , Cholesterol 132 mg , Sodium 1270 mg , Total Carbs 25.5 g , Fiber 3.9 g , Sugar 13 g , Protein 36.4 g

American Chop Suey

Preparation time: 15 minutes
Cooking time: 35 minutes
Total time: 50 minutes
Servings: 6

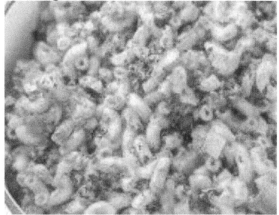

Ingredients:

- 1 tablespoon canola oil
- 1 lb uncooked ground beef
- 1 red bell pepper, chopped
- 1 onion, chopped
- 16-ounce uncooked elbow macaroni
- 24-ounce pasta sauce
- 4 cups of water
- ¼ cup Worcestershire sauce
- ½ teaspoon black pepper
- ¼ teaspoon kosher salt

How to prepare:

1. Turn on the Ninja Foodi and select sauté.
2. Add in oil and sauté for 2 minutes.
3. Add in remaining ingredients and close the lid.
4. Select "bake/roast" for 33 minutes.
5. Open the lid and serve.

Nutritional Values:

Calories 564 , Total Fat 11.3 g , Saturated Fat 3 g , Cholesterol 70 mg , Sodium 732 mg , Total Carbs 77.4 g , Fiber 6.1 g , Sugar 15.8 g , Protein 35.2 g

Chicken Spinach Noodle Bake

Preparation time: 15 minutes
Cooking time: 30 minutes
Total time: 45 minutes
Servings: 6

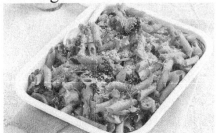

Ingredients:

- 1½ lbs chicken breasts, uncooked, boneless, skinless and cubed
- 3½ cups water
- 1 pound uncooked elbow pasta
- 1 pound whole-milk ricotta cheese
- 1½ cups shredded mozzarella cheese
- 3 garlic cloves, minced
- 4 cups baby spinach
- 1 teaspoon salt

How to prepare:

1. Place all ingredients in the pot and stir well.
2. Close the lid and select "bake/roast."
3. Set timer to 30 minutes.
4. Open the lid and serve.

Nutritional Values:

Calories 803 , Total Fat 12.4 g , Saturated Fat 3.1 g , Cholesterol 105 mg , Sodium 562 mg , Total Carbs 113.5 g , Fiber 5.8 g , Sugar 5.4 g , Protein 54.2 g

Shrimp Scampi

Preparation time: 10 minutes
Cooking time: 35 minutes
Total time: 45 minutes
Servings: 4

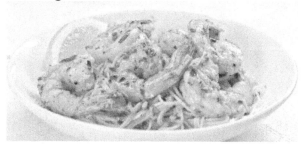

Ingredients:

- 4 tablespoons butter
- 4 cloves garlic, minced
- ¼ teaspoon crush red pepper
- 1 cup parsley, chopped
- Salt to taste
- Black pepper to taste
- ½ cup dry white wine
- 4 cups of water
- 1 pound angel hair pasta, broken in half
- 1 lb shrimp, frozen cooked, peeled

How to prepare:

1. Place butter in the pot and select sauté.
2. Let butter melt and add all ingredients except shrimps.
3. Cook for 5 minutes and close the lid.
4. Select "bake/roast" for 15 minutes at 300 degrees F.
5. Open the lid and in shrimps and select sauté.
6. Cook for 10 minutes until shrimps are tender and heated.
7. Serve and enjoy.

Nutritional Values:

Calories 598 , Total Fat 16.2 g , Saturated Fat 8.3 g , Cholesterol 352 mg , Sodium 444 mg , Total Carbs 66.6 g , Fiber 0.6 g , Sugar 0.4 g , Protein 39.4 g

Spaghetti Meatballs

Preparation time: 10 minutes
Cooking time: 25 minutes
Total time: 35 minutes
Servings: 4

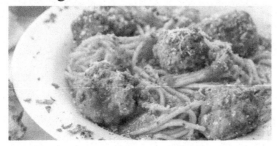

Ingredients:

- 4 cups of water
- 1 pound spaghetti, broken in half
- 24 ounces pasta sauce
- 24 lbs frozen meatballs

How to prepare:

1. Add all ingredients in the pot and mix well.
2. Close the lid and select "bake/roast."
3. Set timer for 25 minutes at 300 degrees F.
4. Open the lid, mix well and serve.

Nutritional Values:

Calories 655 , Total Fat 19.2 g , Saturated Fat 5.1 g , Cholesterol 161 mg , Sodium 1104 mg , Total Carbs 87.5 g , Fiber 4.4 g , Sugar 16 g , Protein 31.9 g

Chicken Parmesan with Penne

Preparation time: 10 minutes
Cooking time: 22 minutes
Total time: 32 minutes
Servings: 4

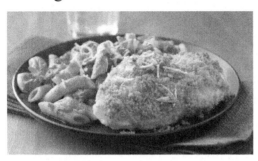

Ingredients:

- 1 pound penne pasta, uncooked
- 4 cups of water
- 4 teaspoons kosher salt, divided
- 4 chicken cutlets, uncooked
- 2 eggs, beaten
- 1 cup all-purpose flour
- 1 cup seasoned bread crumbs
- ½ cup parmesan cheese, grated
- 24 ounces marinara sauce, ¼ cup reserved
- 2 tablespoons olive oil
- 1 bunch broccolini
- 1 cup mozzarella cheese

How to prepare:

1. Add water, 2 teaspoons salt and pasta in the pot.
2. Close the lid and select "pressure."
3. Set the timer to 2 minutes at "high."
4. While pasta is cooking, take a bowl.
5. Add flour, salt and combine.
6. Take another bowl, add eggs, 2 tablespoons water and combine.
7. Take the third bowl and add parmesan and crumbs in it. Mix well.
8. Firstly cover chicken in flour, then in eggs and then with crumbs.
9. Repeat till all chicken is covered and set aside.
10. When pasta is cooked, do a quick release.
11. Open the lid and add marinara sauce, reserving ¼ cup.
12. Add in broccolini and mix well.

13. Place chicken on trivet and trivet in the pot.
14. Close the lid and select "air crisp."
15. Set the timer to 15 minutes at 325 degrees F.
16. Open the lid take pour remaining sauce over chicken.
17. Close the lid, select "broil" and set the timer to 5 minutes.
18. Open the lid, serve and enjoy.

Nutritional Values:

Calories 1103 , Total Fat 31.2 g , Saturated Fat 7.9 g , Cholesterol 305 mg , Sodium 3819 mg , Total Carbs 130.4 g , Fiber 6.7 g , Sugar 17 g , Protein 71.5 g

Rice Recipes

Chicken and Rice

Preparation time: 15 minutes
Cooking time: 33 minutes
Total time: 48 minutes
Servings: 6

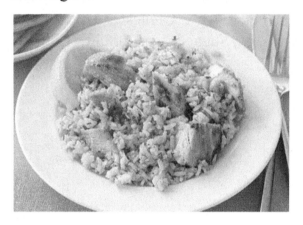

Ingredients:
- 2 tablespoons extra virgin olive oil
- 1 pound mushrooms, cleaned and sliced
- 2 cups brown rice
- ½ cup white wine
- 2 cups chicken stock
- 1¾ lbs chicken thighs, boneless and skinless
- 1 tablespoon kosher salt
- 2 teaspoons smoked paprika
- 2 teaspoons granulated garlic
- 2 teaspoons onion powder
- 1 teaspoon dried thyme
- ½ teaspoon ground white pepper
- 1/8 teaspoon cayenne pepper

How to prepare:
1. Select sauté and let pot heat for 5 minutes.
2. Add in oil, mushrooms and sauté for 5 minutes, stirring continuously.
3. Add in remaining ingredients and stir to combine.
4. Close the lid and select "pressure."
5. Set the timer to 22 minutes at "high."
6. Do a natural release for 10 minutes and then a quick release.

7. Open the lid and serve.

Nutritional Values:

Calories 384 , Total Fat 11.9 g , Saturated Fat 2.5 g , Cholesterol 28 mg , Sodium 1451 mg , Total Carbs 53.5 g , Fiber 3.4 g , Sugar 2.3 g , Protein 13.6 g

Paella

Preparation time: 10 minutes
Cooking time: 12 minutes
Total time: 22 minutes
Servings: 8

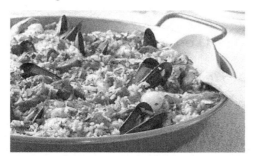

Ingredients:

- 3 tablespoons olive oil
- 4 chorizo, sliced
- 4 chicken thighs, cubed and skinless
- 1 onion, finely chopped
- 1 red bell pepper, chopped
- 3 garlic cloves, minced
- 1½ teaspoons paprika
- 1 teaspoon dried oregano
- ½ teaspoon crushed red pepper
- 1 teaspoon kosher salt
- ½ teaspoon pepper
- 1 can diced tomatoes
- ½ cup white wine
- ¾ cup chicken stock
- 1½ cups basmati rice
- 1 lb shrimp, frozen

How to prepare:

1. Select sauté and let pot heat for 5 minutes.
2. Add in oil, chicken, sausage and cook for 5 minutes.
3. Add in onion, red pepper, garlic, spices and sauté for 5 minutes.
4. Add in remaining ingredients and close the lid.
5. Select "pressure" and timer to 2 minutes at high.
6. Do a quick release.
7. Open the lid and serve.

.

Nutritional Values:
Calories 890 , Total Fat 24.4 g , Saturated Fat 7.1 g , Cholesterol 211 mg , Sodium 945 mg , Total Carbs 109.2 g , Fiber 3.4 g , Sugar 3 g , Protein 51.4 g

Kimchi Fried Rice

Preparation time: 10 minutes
Cooking time: 12 minutes
Total time: 24 minutes
Servings: 4

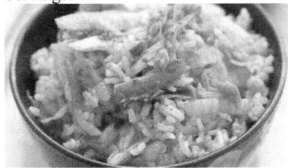

Ingredients:

- 2 tablespoons canola oil
- 1/2 onion, peeled, chopped
- 1 clove garlic, peeled, chopped
- 1 cup basmati rice
- 1/2 cup kimchi, chopped
- 3/4 cup frozen peas and carrots
- 1 1/2 cups chicken stock
- 2 tablespoons soy sauce
- 4 eggs, lightly beaten

How to prepare:

1. Select sauté and let pot heat for 5 minutes.
2. Add in oil, onion, garlic and sauté for 3 minutes.
3. Add in rice, kimchi, stock, vegetables, soy sauce and close the lid.
4. Select "pressure," set the timer to 4 minutes at "high."
5. Do a natural release for 10 minutes and then a quick release.
6. Open the lid and select sauté.
7. Pour in eggs and stir well until they began to scramble.
8. Close the lid and select "air crisp."
9. Set time to 6 minutes at 400 degrees F, after 3 minutes open lid and stir rice and then resume.
10. When time is over, open the lid and serve.

Nutritional Values:

Calories 324 , Total Fat 12 g , Saturated Fat 2 g , Cholesterol 164 mg , Sodium 865 mg , Total Carbs 43 g , Fiber 1.9 g , Sugar 2.7 g , Protein 10.7 g

Rice Pilaf

Preparation time: 15 minutes
Cooking time: 14 minutes
Total time: 29 minutes
Servings: 4

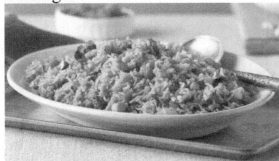

Ingredients:

- 1 box rice pilaf
- 1 3/4 cups water
- 1 tablespoon butter
- 4 carrots, peeled, cut in half, lengthwise
- 4 uncooked boneless skin-on chicken thighs
- 2 tablespoons honey, warmed
- 1/2 teaspoon smoked paprika
- 1/2 teaspoon ground cumin
- 2 teaspoons kosher salt, divided
- 1 tablespoon extra virgin olive oil
- 2 teaspoons poultry spice

How to prepare:

1. Place all the ingredients in the pot and close the lid.
2. Select "pressure" and set timer 4 minutes at "high."
3. Do a quick release.
4. Select "broil" and broil for 10 minutes.
5. Open the lid and serve.

Nutritional Values:

Calories 392 , Total Fat 17.3 g , Saturated Fat 5.3 g , Cholesterol 138 mg , Sodium 1357 mg , Total Carbs 15 g , Fiber 1.7 g , Sugar 11.7 g , Protein 42.9 g

Rice and Chicken with Yogurt Herb Sauce

Preparation time: 10 minutes
Cooking time: 23 minutes
Total time: 33 minutes
Servings: 8

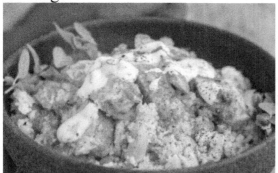

Ingredients:

- 2 pounds boneless skinless chicken thighs, cut in 1-inch pieces
- 1 packet (1 ounce) mild taco seasoning
- 1 bag (16 ounces) frozen mixed vegetables
- 2 cans (10 ounces each) enchilada sauce
- 1 cup of water
- 2 cups uncooked jasmine rice

Herb Sauce:

- 1 cup Greek yogurt
- 1/2 jalapeño pepper, seeds removed, finely chopped
- 1/4 cup fresh cilantro, minced
- 1/4 cup fresh mint, minced
- 2 tablespoons olive oil
- Juice of 1/2 lime

How to prepare:

1. Select sauté and let pot heat for 3 minutes.
2. Add in chicken, seasoning and let meat brown for 10 minutes. Stir occasionally.
3. Add in vegetables, sauce, water, rice and close the lid.
4. Select "pressure" for 2 minutes at "high."
5. Do a natural release for 10 minutes and then a quick release.
6. Meanwhile, take a bowl and stir all sauce ingredients in it.
7. Open the lid, serve and top with sauce.

Nutritional Values:

Calories 644 , Total Fat 14.8 g , Saturated Fat 3.9 g , Cholesterol 102 mg , Sodium 167 mg , Total Carbs 90.7 g , Fiber 23.5 g , Sugar 3.3 g , Protein 47.8 g

Lime Cilantro Cauliflower rice

Preparation time: 10 minutes
Cooking time: 10 minutes
Total time: 20 minutes
Servings: 3

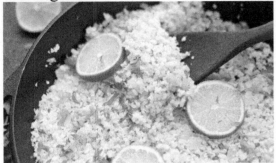

Ingredients:

- 1 small head cauliflower, cut in florets
- 2 cloves garlic, peeled
- ½ cup cilantro
- 2 tablespoons olive oil
- 4 tablespoons lemon juice
- 1 tablespoon salt

How to prepare:

1. Add cauliflower, garlic, cilantro in a blender and blend.
2. Turn on Ninja Foodi and select sauté.
3. Add in olive oil and heat it for 1 minute.
4. Add in cauliflower mixture and cook for 7 minutes. Stir continuously.
5. Add salt, lime juice and mix well.
6. Serve and enjoy.

Nutritional Values:

Calories 111 , Total Fat 9.6 g , Saturated Fat 1.5 g , Cholesterol 0 mg , Sodium 2358 mg , Total Carbs 5.9 g , Fiber 2.4 g , Sugar 2.6 g , Protein 2.1 g

Cauliflower Fried Rice

Preparation time: 10 minutes
Cooking time: 8 minutes
Total time: 18 minutes
Servings: 4

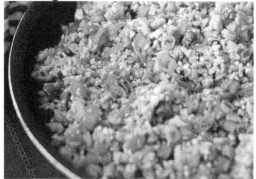

Ingredients:

- 3 cups cauliflower florets
- 1 medium carrot, peeled, cut in 1-inch pieces
- 1-inch piece fresh ginger, peeled
- 2 tablespoons sesame oil
- 2 green onions, chopped
- 1/2 cup peas
- 2 tablespoons soy sauce
- 1/4 teaspoon ground black pepper

How to prepare:

1. Place cauliflower in a precision processor and chop until desired consistency has reached.
2. Place carrot and ginger into precision processor and chop.
3. Turn on Ninja Foodi and select sauté.
4. Add in oil and let it heat for 1 minute.
5. Add in chopped vegetables and sauté for 5 minutes.
6. Add in remaining ingredients and cook for 2 minutes.
7. Serve and enjoy.

Nutritional Values:

Calories 124 , Total Fat 8.7 g , Saturated Fat 1.2 g , Cholesterol 0 mg , Sodium 579 mg , Total Carbs 9.6 g , Fiber 3.5 g , Sugar 3.9 g , Protein 3.5 g

Fajita Rice Bowl

Preparation time: 10 minutes
Cooking time: 47 minutes
Total time: 57 minutes
Servings: 6

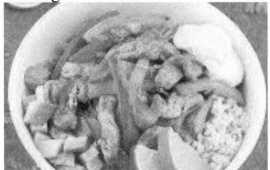

Ingredients:

- 1 tablespoon canola oil
- 1 1/2 pounds uncooked beef flank steak, cut in 2-inch x 1/4-inch slices
- 2 packets (1.25 ounces each) fajita seasoning mix
- 2 bell peppers, thinly sliced
- 1 medium onion, peeled, thinly sliced
- 2 1/2 cups low-sodium beef broth
- 1 cup uncooked long grain white rice

How to prepare:

1. Select sauté and let the pot heat for 5 minutes.
2. Add oil and heat it for 2 minutes.
3. Add in all ingredients, except rice and broth.
4. Cook for 10 minutes, stirring continuously.
5. Add in rice and broth.
6. Cover the lid, select "pressure."
7. Set the timer to 30 minutes at "low."
8. Open the lid, stir and serve.

Nutritional Values:

Calories 384 , Total Fat 10.3 g , Saturated Fat 3.1 g , Cholesterol 101 mg , Sodium 471 mg , Total Carbs 30.6 g , Fiber 1.3 g , Sugar 3.1 g , Protein 39.3 g

Spanish Rice

Preparation time: 10 minutes
Cooking time: 12 minutes
Total time: 22 minutes
Servings: 4

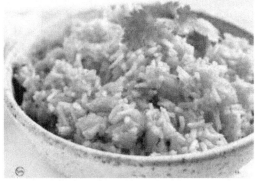

Ingredients:

- 1 pound ground beef
- 1 small onion chopped
- 1 chopped green pepper chopped
- 1 garlic clove, minced
- 1 tablespoon chili powder
- 2 Cups tomato or vegetable juice
- 1 cup uncooked long grain rice
- 1/2 teaspoon salt

How to prepare:

1. Turn on the Ninja Foodi and select sauté.
2. Add all ingredients and stir well.
3. Close the lid and select "pressure."
4. Set the timer to 12 minutes at "low."
5. Do a quick release, open lid and serve.

Nutritional Values:

Calories 416 , Total Fat 8 g , Saturated Fat 2.9 g , Cholesterol 101 mg , Sodium 393 mg , Total Carbs 44.8 g , Fiber 3.2 g , Sugar 4 g , Protein 39.2 g

Hainanese Chicken Rice

Preparation time: 15 minutes
Cooking time: 15 minutes
Total time: 30 minutes
Servings: 4

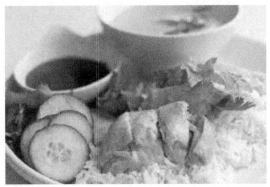

Ingredients:

- 1 cup basmati rice, drained and rinsed
- 1 cup of water
- 1 pound chicken thighs boneless, bite size
- 1 pack Asian Gourmet Hainanese Chicken Rice Mix

How to prepare:

1. Place all the ingredients in the Ninja Foodi.
2. Close the lid and select «pressure.»
3. Set the timer to 6 minutes at "high."
4. Do a natural release, open the lid and serve.

Nutritional Values:

Calories 169 , Total Fat 0.3 g , Saturated Fat 0.1 g , Cholesterol 0 mg , Sodium 4 mg , Total Carbs 37 g , Fiber 0.6 g , Sugar 0.1 g , Protein 3.4 g

Savoury Beef & Lamb Recipes

Lemon Flank Steak

Preparation time: 10 minutes
Cooking time: 16 minutes
Total time: 26 minutes
Servings: 4

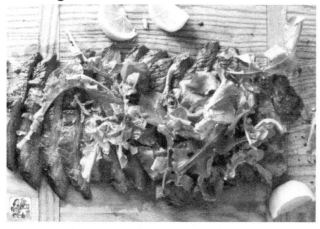

Ingredients:

- 1 tablespoon butter
- 1 tablespoon fresh thyme, chopped
- 4 grass fed flank steaks
- 2 tablespoons lemon juice
- Salt to taste
- Pepper to taste

How to prepare:

1. Turn on the Ninja Foodi and select sauté.
2. Add butter and select "start" and cook for 3 minutes.
3. Add steak and cook for 3 minutes on each side.
4. Press "stop" and stir in remaining ingredients.
5. Close the lid and set the valve to seal.
6. Set the Ninja Foodi to "Manual" at high pressure for 10 minutes, release the pressure quickly.
7. Open the lid and serve.

Nutritional Values:

Calories 359 , Total Fat 17.1 g , Saturated Fat 7.8 g , Cholesterol 34 mg , Sodium 456 mg , Total Carbs 0.6 g , Fiber 0.3 g , Sugar0.2 g , Protein 47.5 g

Creamy Beef Steak

Preparation time: 1 hour 15 minutes
Cooking time: 30 minutes
Total time: 1 hour 45 minutes
Servings: 6

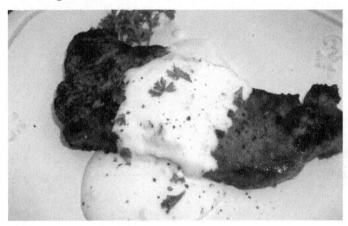

Ingredients:

- ½ cup butter
- 4 garlic cloves, minced
- 2 pounds beef top sirloin steaks
- Salt and black pepper, to taste
- 1½ cup cream

How to prepare:

1. Rub beef steaks with garlic, salt, and pepper.
2. Marinate beef steaks with butter, cream and set aside.
3. Place grill in the Ninja Foodi and steaks on the grill.
4. Select "broil" and set the timer for 30 minutes at 365 degrees F.
5. Flip steaks in a middle way.

Serve and enjoy.

Nutritional Values:

Calories 353 , Total Fat 24.1 g , Saturated Fat 14.5 g , Cholesterol 113 mg , Sodium 298 mg , Total Carbs 3.9 g , Fiber 0 g , Sugar 1.2 g , Protein 31.8 g

Beef Sirloin Steak

Preparation time: 10 minutes
Cooking time: 17 minutes
Total time: 27 minutes
Servings: 3

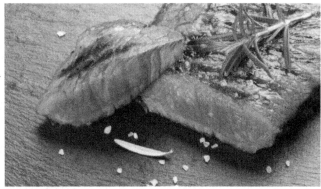

Ingredients:

- 3 tablespoons butter
- ½ teaspoon garlic powder
- 1 pound beef top sirloin steaks
- Salt and black pepper, to taste
- 1 garlic clove, minced

How to prepare:

1. Turn on the Ninja Foodi and select sauté.
2. Add in butter, steaks and sauté for 2 minutes on each side.
3. Add in garlic powder, salt, pepper, and garlic clove.
4. Select "pressure" with a timer for 15 minutes on "Md: Hi."
5. Serve hot and enjoy.

Nutritional Values:

Calories 246 , Total Fat 13.1 g , Saturated Fat 7.6 g , Cholesterol 81mg , Sodium 224 mg , Total Carbs 2 g , Fiber 0.1 g , Sugar0.1 g , Protein 31.3 g

Lamb Chops

Preparation time: 15 minutes
Cooking time: 42 minutes
Total time: 57 minutes
Servings: 4

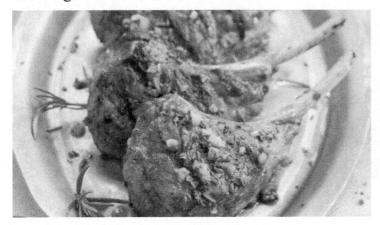

Ingredients:

- 4 tablespoons butter
- 3 tablespoons lemon juice
- 4 lamb chops, bone-in
- 2 tablespoons almond flour
- 1 cup picante sauce

How to prepare:

1. Do a coating of almond flour on the chops and set aside.
2. Turn on the Ninja Foodi and select sauté.
3. Add in butter, chops and sauté for 2 minutes.
4. Stir in picante sauce and lemon juice.
5. Close the lid.
6. Select "pressure" and set a timer for 40 minutes at "Hi."
7. Release the pressure quickly, open lid and serve.

Nutritional Values:

Calories 284 , Total Fat 19.5 g , Saturated Fat 9.7 g , Cholesterol 107 mg , Sodium 150 mg , Total Carbs 1 g , Fiber 0.4 g , Sugar 0.3 g , Protein 24.8 g

Lamb Roast

Preparation time: 15 minutes
Cooking time: 60 minutes
Total time: 1 hour 15 minutes
Servings: 6

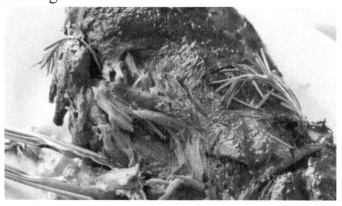

Ingredients:

- 2 pounds lamb roasted Wegmans
- 1 cup onion soup
- 1 cups beef broth
- Salt and black pepper, to taste

How to prepare:

1. Place lamb roast in the pot of Ninja Foodi.
2. Add in onion soup, salt, pepper, beef broth.
3. Close the lid and select "pressure."
4. Set timer for 55 minutes at "Md: Hi."
5. Release pressure naturally, dish out and serve.

Nutritional Values:

Calories 349 , Total Fat 18.8 g , Saturated Fat 0.2 g , Cholesterol 122 mg , Sodium 480 mg , Total Carbs 2.9 g , Fiber 0.3 g , Sugar 1.2 g , Protein 39.9 g

Indian Classical Beef

Preparation time: 10 minutes
Cooking time: 20 minutes
Total time: 30minutes
Servings: 4

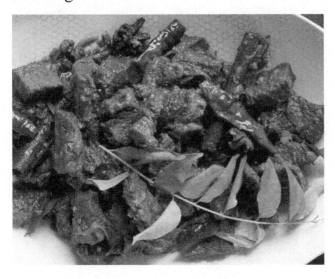

Ingredients:
- ½ yellow onion, chopped
- 1 tablespoon olive oil
- 2 garlic cloves, minced
- 1 jalapeño pepper, chopped
- 1 cup cherry tomatoes, quartered
- 1 teaspoon fresh lemon juice
- 1 pound grass-fed ground beef
- 1 pound fresh collard greens, trimmed and chopped

Spices
- 1 teaspoon ground cumin
- ½ teaspoon ground ginger
- 1 teaspoon ground coriander
- ½ teaspoon ground fennel seeds
- ½ teaspoon ground cinnamon
- Salt and black pepper, to taste
- ½ teaspoon ground turmeric

How to prepare:
1. Turn on the Ninja Foodi and select sauté.
2. Add onions, garlic and sauté for 3 minutes.

3. Add jalapeno peppers, beef, spices and close the lid.
4. Select "pressure" with a timer of 15 minutes at "Md: Hi."
5. Release pressure naturally and open the lid.
6. Add cherry tomatoes, collard greens and sauté for 3 minutes.
7. Stir in lemon juice, black pepper, salt, dish out and serve.

Nutritional Values:
Calories 409 , Total Fat 16.5 g , Saturated Fat 8 g , Cholesterol 158 mg , Sodium 769 mg , Total Carbs 5.7 g , Fiber 0.6 g , Sugar 1.9 g , Protein 56.4 g

Steak Meal

Preparation time: 15 minutes
Cooking time: 27 minutes
Total time: 42 minutes
Servings: 4

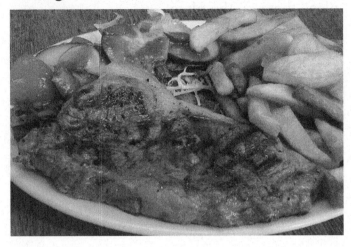

Ingredients:
For Steak Sauce:
- 2 tablespoons yellow onion
- 2 tablespoons butter
- 2 garlic cloves, minced
- 1½ cups homemade beef broth
- ¾ cup fresh blueberries
- 1 teaspoon fresh thyme, chopped finely
- 2 tablespoons fresh lemon juice

For Steak:
- 4 (6-ounce) grass-fed flank steaks
- 1 tablespoon butter
- Salt and black pepper, to taste
- How to prepare:

For Sauce:
1. Turn on the Ninja Foodi and select sauté.
2. Add butter, garlic, thyme, onions and sauté for 3 minutes.
3. Stir in broth and close the lid.
4. Select "pressure" with a timer of 10 minutes on "Md: Low.
5. Release pressure naturally and open the lid.
6. Stir in blueberries, lemon juice, salt, and black pepper.
7. Select sauté and sauté for 2 minutes, transfer it in a bowl.

For Steak:
1. Turn on the Ninja Foodi and select sauté.
2. Add in steaks, butter, salt, pepper and sauté for 2 minutes.
3. Lock the lid and select "pressure."
4. Set timer for 10 minutes at "Md: Hi."
5. Release the pressure naturally and place them on the plate.
6. Pour sauce over steaks and enjoy.

Nutritional Values:
Calories 409 , Total Fat 16.5 g , Saturated Fat 8 g , Cholesterol 158 mg , Sodium 769 mg , Total Carbs 5.7 g , Fiber 0.6 g , Sugar 1.9 g , Protein 56.4 g

Zesty Meatloaf

Preparation time: 15 minutes
Cooking time: 1 hour 10 minutes
Total time: 1 hour 25 minutes
Servings: 6

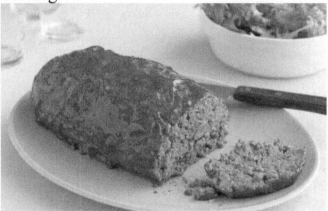

Ingredients:

- ½ cup onion, chopped
- 2 garlic cloves, minced
- ¼ cup sugar-free ketchup
- 1 pound grass-fed lean ground beef
- ½ cup green bell pepper, seeded and chopped
- 1 cup cheddar cheese, grated
- 2 organic eggs, beaten
- 1 teaspoon dried thyme, crushed
- 3 cups fresh spinach, chopped
- 6 cups mozzarella cheese, freshly grated
- Black pepper, to taste

How to prepare:

1. Take a bowl and add all ingredients in it except spinach and cheese.
2. Mix well so they can combine well.
3. Place a wax paper on a smooth surface and arrange meat on it.
4. Top it with cheese, spinach and roll it up around mixture to form a meatloaf.
5. Remove wax paper and place meatloaf in Ninja Foodis pot.
6. Select "bake/roast" with a timer of 70 minutes at 380 degrees F.
7. Dish out and serve.

Nutritional Values:

Calories 223 , Total Fat 14.5 g , Saturated Fat 8.2 g , Cholesterol 102mg , Sodium 338 mg , Total Carbs 4.2 g , Fiber 0.8 g , Sugar 1.2 g , Protein 19.1 g

Beef Fajitas

Preparation time: 10 minutes
Cooking time: 7 hours 3minutes
Total time: 7 hours 13 minutes
Servings: 8

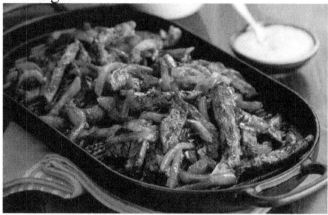

Ingredients:

- 2 tablespoons butter
- 2 bell peppers, sliced
- 2 pounds beef, sliced
- 2 tablespoons fajita seasoning
- 2 onions, sliced

How to prepare:

1. Turn on the Ninja Foodi and select sauté.
2. Add in all ingredients and sauté for 3 minutes.
3. Select "slow cooker" and cook for 7 hours.
4. Dish out and serve.

Nutritional Values:

Calories 353 , Total Fat 13.4 g , Saturated Fat 6 g , Cholesterol 145 mg , Sodium 304 mg , Total Carbs 8.5 g , Fiber 1.3 g , Sugar3.6 g , Protein 46.7 g

Taco Casserole

Preparation time: 5 minutes
Cooking time: 25 minutes
Total time: 30 minutes
Servings: 6

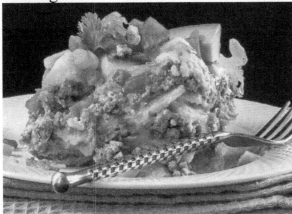

Ingredients:

- 1 cup cheddar cheese, shredded
- 1 cup cottage cheese
- 2 pounds ground beef
- 1 cup of salsa
- 2 tablespoons taco seasoning

How to prepare:

1. Take a bowl and mix taco seasoning with beef.
2. Add in salsa, cheddar and cottage cheese and mix well.
3. Place this mixture in the pot of Ninja Foodi and close the lid.
4. Select "bake/roast" with a timer of 25 minutes at 370 degrees F.
5. Open the lid and serve immediately.

Nutritional Values:

Calories 416 , Total Fat 16.5 g , Saturated Fat 8 g , Cholesterol 158 mg , Sodium 910 mg , Total Carbs 7 g , Fiber 0.7 g , Sugar 2.2 g , Protein 56.4 g

Flavorful Chicken & Poultry Recipes

Creamy Chicken Fillets

Preparation time: 15 minutes
Cooking time: 15 minutes
Total time: 30 minutes
Servings: 4

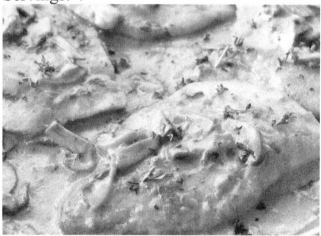

Ingredients:

- 1 small onion
- 2 tablespoons butter
- 1 pound chicken breasts
- ½ cup sour cream
- Salt, to taste

How to prepare:

1. Season chicken with salt, pepper and set aside.
2. Turn on the Ninja Foodi and select sauté.
3. Add in butter, onions an sauté for 3 minutes.
4. Add chicken breasts and close the lid.
5. Cook for 10 minutes on sauté mode and open the lid.
6. Stir in sour cream and cook for 4 minutes.
7. Stir gently, serve and enjoy.

Nutritional Values:

Calories 447 , Total Fat 26.9 g , Saturated Fat 12.9 g , Cholesterol 172 mg , Sodium 206 mg , Total Carbs 3.8 g , Fiber 0.5 g , Sugar 1.1 g , Protein 45.3 g

Chicken Ropa Vieja

Preparation time: 10 minutes
Cooking time: 4 hours 8 minutes
Total time: 4 hours 18 minutes
Servings: 8

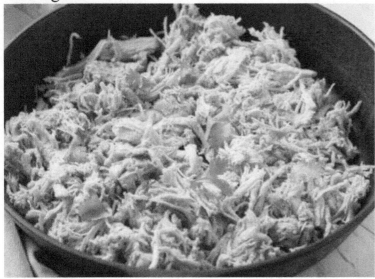

Ingredients:

- 3 tablespoons butter
- ½ yellow onion, sliced into long strips
- 1 tablespoon tomato paste
- 1/8 teaspoon red pepper flakes
- 1½ pounds chicken pieces, boneless and skinless
- ½ tablespoon oregano
- ½ red bell pepper, sliced into long strips
- 3 garlic cloves, minced
- ½ teaspoon cumin powder
- ½ green bell pepper, sliced into long strips
- Salt and black pepper, to taste
- ½ cup tomatoes, diced

How to prepare:

1. Season chicken with cumin powder, oregano, black pepper, salt, and red pepper.
2. Turn on the Ninja Foodi and select sauté.
3. Add in butter, seasoned chicken and sauté for 2 minutes.
4. Add in onions, bell peppers and sauté for 1 minute.
5. Add diced tomatoes, tomato paste, garlic and give a stir.
6. Lock the lid and select "slow cooker" keeping it on high for 4 hours.
7. Open the lid and break chicken pieces by stirring.

8. Select "air crisp" and cook for 5 minutes at 360 degrees F.
9. Serve and enjoy.

Nutritional Values:

Calories 285 , Total Fat 11.2 g , Saturated Fat 5.5 g , Cholesterol 122 mg , Sodium 182 mg , Total Carbs 6 g , Fiber 1.4 g , Sugar 3 g , Protein 40.6 g

Stuffed Whole Chicken

Preparation time: 15 minutes
Cooking time: 8 hours
Total time: 8 hours 15 minutes
Servings: 6

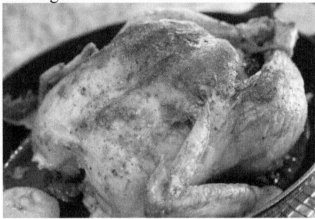

Ingredients:

- 1 cup mozzarella cheese
- 4 whole garlic cloves, peeled
- 1 (2-pound) whole chicken, cleaned, pat dried
- Salt and black pepper, to taste
- 2 tablespoons fresh lemon juice

How to prepare:

1. Stuff chicken with mozzarella cheese and garlic cloves.
2. Season it with salt and pepper.
3. Place chicken in Ninja Foodi and pour lemon juice over it.
4. Select "slow cooker" and cook for 8 hours.
5. Dish out and serve.

Nutritional Values:

Calories 309 , Total Fat 12.1 g , Saturated Fat 3.6 g , Cholesterol 137 mg , Sodium 201 mg , Total Carbs 1.6 g , Fiber 0.8 g , Sugar 0.7 g , Protein 45.8 g

Stuffed Turkey Rolls

Preparation time: 5 minutes
Cooking time: 20 minutes
Total time: 25 minutes
Servings: 8

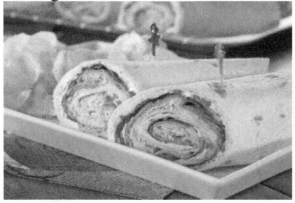

Ingredients:

- 4 tablespoons fresh sage leaves
- 8 ham slices
- 8 (6-ounce) turkey cutlets
- Salt and black pepper, to taste
- 2 tablespoons butter, melted

How to prepare:

1. Season turkey cutlets with pepper and salt.
2. Roll cutlets and wrap each one with ham slices.
3. Coat each roll with butter and wrap with sage leaves over each cutlet.
4. Select "bake/roast" and add rolls in Ninja Foodi and bake for 10 minutes at 360 degrees F.
5. Dish out and serve.

Nutritional Values:

Calories 467 , Total Fat 24.8 g , Saturated Fat 10 g , Cholesterol 218 mg , Sodium 534 mg , Total Carbs 1.7 g , Fiber 0.8 g , Sugar 0 g , Protein 56 g

Creamy Tasty Turkey Breasts

Preparation time: 15 minutes
Cooking time: 2 hours
Total time: 2 hours 15 minutes
Servings: 6

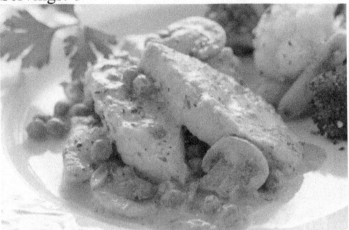

Ingredients:

- 1½ cups Italian dressing
- 2 garlic cloves, minced
- 1 (2-pound) bone-in turkey breast
- 2 tablespoons butter
- Salt and black pepper, to taste

How to prepare:

1. Take a bowl and add garlic cloves, salt, pepper and mix well.
2. Season turkey with this mixture.
3. Grease pot of Ninja Foodi with butter and place turkey breasts in it.
4. Top with Italian dressing.
5. Select "bake/roast" and set the timer for 2 hours at 330 degrees F.
6. Dish out and serve.

Nutritional Values:

Calories 369 , Total Fat 23.2 g , Saturated Fat 5.1 g , Cholesterol 104 mg , Sodium 990 mg , Total Carbs 6.5 g , Fiber 0 g , Sugar 4.9 g , Protein 35.4 g

Hasselback Chicken

Preparation time: 15 minutes
Cooking time: 1 hour
Total time: 1 hour 15 minutes
Servings: 8

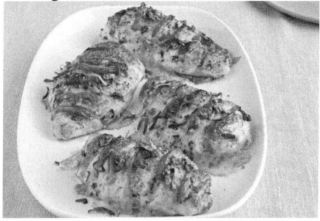

Ingredients:

- 4 tablespoons butter
- Salt and black pepper, to taste
- 2 cups fresh mozzarella cheese, thinly sliced
- 8 large chicken breasts
- 4 large Roma tomatoes, thinly sliced

How to prepare:

1. Make deep cuts in chicken and season it with salt and pepper.
2. Stuff mozzarella cheese and tomatoes in these cuts.
3. Grease pot of Ninja Foodi with butter.
4. Add in chicken breasts and select "bake/roast."
5. Set timer for 1 hour at 365 degrees F.
6. Dish out and serve.

Nutritional Values:

Calories 287 , Total Fat 15 g , Saturated Fat 6.6 g , Cholesterol 112 mg , Sodium 178 mg , Total Carbs 3.8 g , Fiber 1.1 g , Sugar 2.4 g , Protein 33.2 g

Turkey Cutlets

Preparation time: 15 minutes
Cooking time: 15 minutes
Total time: 30 minutes
Servings: 4

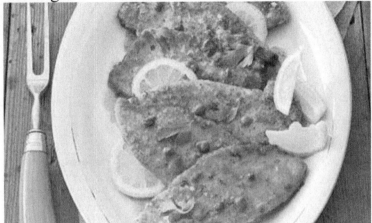

Ingredients:

- 1 teaspoon Greek seasoning
- 1 pound turkey cutlets
- 2 tablespoons olive oil
- 1 teaspoon turmeric powder
- ½ cup almond flour

How to prepare:

1. Take a bowl and add greek seasoning, turmeric powder, almond flour in it. Mix well.
2. Coat turkey cutlets in it and set aside for 30 minutes.
3. Turn on the Ninja Foodi and select sauté.
4. Add oil, turkey cutlets and sauté for 2 minutes.
5. Close the lid.
6. Select "pressure" and set "Lo: Md," cook for 20 minutes.
7. Serve and enjoy.

Nutritional Values:

Calories 340 , Total Fat 19.4 g , Saturated Fat 3.4 g , Cholesterol 86 mg , Sodium 124 mg , Total Carbs 3.7 g , Fiber 1.6 g , Sugar 0 g , Protein 36.3 g

Garlic Turkey Breasts

Preparation time: 15 minutes
Cooking time: 17 minutes
Total time: 32 minutes
Servings: 4

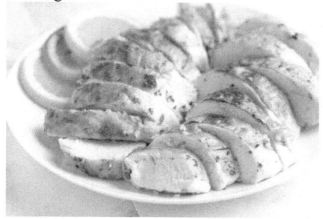

Ingredients:

- ½ teaspoon garlic powder
- 4 tablespoons butter
- ¼ teaspoon dried oregano
- 1 pound turkey breasts, boneless
- 1 teaspoon black pepper
- ½ teaspoon salt
- ¼ teaspoon dried basil

How to prepare:

1. Season turkey on all sides with garlic powder, dried basil, dried oregano, salt, and pepper.
2. Turn on Ninja Foodi and select sauté.
3. Add butter, turkey breasts and sauté for 2 minutes on each side.
4. Close the lid and select "bake/roast."
5. Set timer for 15 minutes at 355 degrees F.
6. Serve and enjoy.

Nutritional Values:

Calories 223 , Total Fat 13.4 g , Saturated Fat 7.7 g , Cholesterol 79 mg , Sodium 1524 mg , Total Carbs 5.4 g , Fiber 0.8 g , Sugar 4.1 g , Protein 19.6 g

Lime Chicken

Preparation time: 5 minutes
Cooking time: 23 minutes
Total time: 28 minutes
Servings: 6

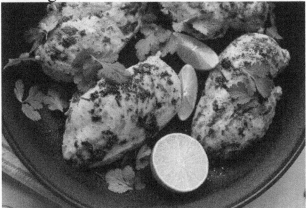

Ingredients:

- ¼ cup cooking wine
- ½ cup organic chicken broth
- 1 onion, diced
- 1 teaspoon of sea salt
- ½ teaspoon paprika
- 5 garlic cloves, minced
- 1 tablespoon lime juice
- ¼ cup butter
- 2 pounds chicken thighs
- 1 teaspoon dried parsley
- 3 green chilies, chopped

How to prepare:

1. Turn on the Ninja Foodi and select sauté.
2. Add in onions, garlic and sauté for 3 minutes.
3. Add in remaining ingredients and close the lid.
4. Select "pressure" and set a timer for 20 minutes at "Md: Hi."
5. Open the lid, dish out and enjoy.

Nutritional Values:

Calories 282 , Total Fat 15.2 g , Saturated Fat 7.2 g , Cholesterol 129 mg , Sodium 2117 mg , Total Carbs 6.3 g , Fiber 0.9 g , Sugar 3.3 g , Protein 27.4 g

Smoky Whole Chicken

Preparation time: 10 minutes
Cooking time: 35 minutes
Total time: 45 minutes
Servings: 5

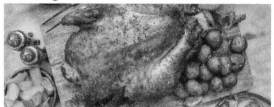

Ingredients:

- 1 teaspoon paprika
- 1 teaspoon garlic powder
- ½ teaspoon onion powder
- Salt to taste
- Pepper to taste
- 1 grass-fed whole chicken, giblets and necks removed
- 1 cup of water
- 1 teaspoon liquid smoke
- 2 tablespoons chicken rub, divided
- Olive oil cooking spray

How to prepare:

1. Take a bowl and mix spices, salt, and pepper.
2. Season chicken with this mixture on all sides.
3. Add 1 cup water, liquid smoke in a pot of Ninja Foodi.
4. Place chicken in cool and crisp basket and this basket in the pot.
5. Close the lid and set the valve to seal position.
6. Set the instant pot to "Manual" at high pressure for 15 minutes, release the pressure quickly through the steam vent.
7. Open the lid of the Ninja Foodi and spray chicken with oil.
8. Season chicken with chicken rub.
9. Close the lid again and select "air crisps."
10. Set timer for 10 minutes at 400 degrees F.
11. Open the lid and serve.

Nutritional Values:

Calories 58 , Total Fat 2.9 g , Saturated Fat 1 g , Cholesterol 16 mg , Sodium 297 mg , Total Carbs 2.4 g , Fiber 0.2 g , Sugar 0.3 g , Protein 4.4 g

Great Pork Recipes

Bacon Pork Chops

Preparation time: 10 minutes
Cooking time: 18 minutes
Total time: 28 minutes
Servings: 4

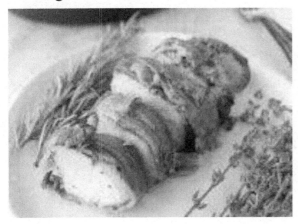

Ingredients:

- ½ cup Swiss cheese, shredded
- 4 pork chops, bone-in
- 6 bacon strips, cut in half
- Salt and black pepper, to taste
- 1 tablespoon butter

How to prepare:

1. Season pork chops with pepper and salt.
2. Turn on Ninja Foodi and select sauté.
3. Add butter, pork chops and sauté for 3 minutes on each side.
4. Add cheese and bacon strips.
5. Close the lid and select "pressure."
6. Set timer to 15 minutes on "Medium Low."
7. Transfer steaks in serving plate and serve.

Nutritional Values:

Calories 483 , Total Fat 40 g , Saturated Fat 16.2 g , Cholesterol 89 mg , Sodium 552 mg , Total Carbs 0.7 g , Fiber 0 g , Sugar 0.2 g , Protein 27.7 g

Jamaican Jerk Pork Roast

Preparation time: 15 minutes
Cooking time: 23 minutes
Total time: 38 minutes
Servings: 3

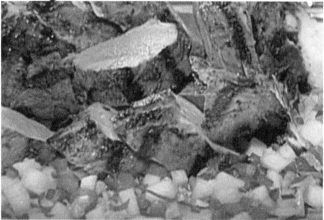

Ingredients:

- 1 tablespoon butter
- 1/8 cup beef broth
- 1 pound pork shoulder
- 1/8 cup Jamaican jerk spice blend

How to prepare:

1. Season pork with Jamaican jerk spice.
2. Turn on the Ninja Foodi and select sauté.
3. Add butter, seasoned pork and sauté for 3 minutes
4. Close the lid and press "pressure."
5. Set the timer for 20 minutes on low and release pressure naturally.
6. Serve and enjoy.

Nutritional Values:

Calories 477 , Total Fat 36.2 g , Saturated Fat 14.3 g , Cholesterol 146 mg , Sodium 162 mg , Total Carbs 0 g , Fiber 0 g , Sugar 0 g , Protein 35.4 g

Pork Carnitas

Preparation time: 15 minutes
Cooking time: 26 minutes
Total time: 41 minutes
Servings: 6

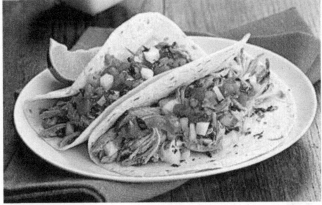

Ingredients:

- 2 tablespoons butter
- 2 oranges, juiced
- 2 pounds pork shoulder, bone-in
- Salt and black pepper, to taste
- 1 teaspoon garlic powder

How to prepare:

1. Season pork with salt and black pepper.
2. Turn on the Ninja Foodi and select sauté.
3. Add in butter, garlic powder and sauté for 1 minute.
4. Add in seasoned pork and sauté for 3 minutes.
5. Stir in orange juice and close the lid.
6. Select "pressure" and set a timer for 15 minutes on "high."
7. Release pressure naturally, open the lid and select "broil."
8. Set timer for 8 minutes at 375 degrees f.
9. Serve and enjoy.

Nutritional Values:

Calories 506 , Total Fat 36.3 g , Saturated Fat 14.3 g , Cholesterol 146 mg , Sodium 130 mg , Total Carbs 7.6 g , Fiber 1.5 g , Sugar 5.8 g , Protein 35.9 g

Mustard Pork Chops

Preparation time: 15 minutes
Cooking time: 30 minutes
Total time: 45 minutes
Servings: 4

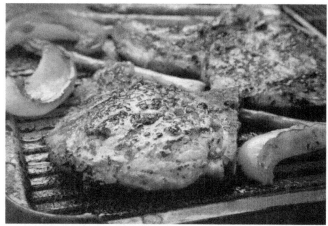

Ingredients:

- 2 tablespoons butter
- 2 tablespoons Dijon mustard
- 4 pork chops
- Salt and black pepper, to taste
- 1 tablespoon fresh rosemary, coarsely chopped

  How to prepare:

1. Marinate chops with Dijon mustard, rosemary, salt, pepper and set aside for 2 hours.
2. Place pork chops, butter in a pot of Ninja Foodi.
3. Close the lid and select "pressure."
4. Set timer for 30 minutes on "Lo: Md."
5. Release pressure naturally, open the lid and serve.

Nutritional Values:

Calories 315 , Total Fat 26.1 g , Saturated Fat 11.2 g , Cholesterol 84 mg , Sodium 186 mg , Total Carbs 1 g , Fiber 0.6 g , Sugar 0.1 g , Protein 18.4 g

Spicy Pork Ribs

Preparation time: 10 minutes
Cooking time: 34 minutes
Total time: 44 minutes
Servings: 4

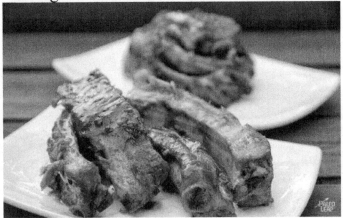

Ingredients:

- 3 lbs pork ribs, cut into thirds
- ¾ cup of water
- 1 tablespoon erythritol
- 1 teaspoon oregano, dried
- 1 teaspoon red chili powder
- ½ teaspoon garlic powder
- ¾ cup tomato paste
- 1 teaspoon dried thyme
- 1 teaspoon sweet paprika
- ½ teaspoon cayenne pepper
- ½ teaspoon onion powder
- Salt to taste
- Pepper to taste

How to prepare:

1. Rub pork ribs with salt, pepper.
2. Place water in the pot of Ninja Foodi.
3. Place ribs in "cook and crisp basket" and place this basket in the pot.
4. Close the lid and set the valve to seal.
5. Select "pressure" and set timer 19 minutes on "high."
6. Quickly release the pressure.
7. Open the lid of the Ninja Foodi.
8. Select "air crisp" and set the timer for 15 minutes at 400 degrees F.
9. Take a bowl and add remaining ingredients in it.

10. Open the lid and coat chops with sauce and close the lid for 5 minutes.
11. Serve and enjoy.

Nutritional Values:

Calories 977 , Total Fat 60.8 g , Saturated Fat 21.6 g , Cholesterol 350 mg , Sodium 293 mg , Total Carbs 13.5 g , Fiber 2.8 g , Sugar 8.8 g , Protein 92.6 g

Pork Chops with Cabbage

Preparation time: 10 minutes
Cooking time: 12 minutes
Total time: 22 minutes
Servings: 6

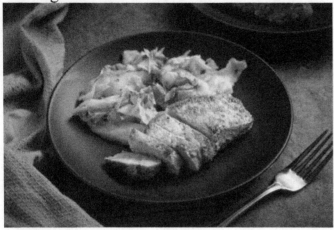

Ingredients:

- 2 lbs pork chops, boneless
- 1 cabbage head, cut in chunks
- ¼ cup butter
- 2 cups chicken broth
- Salt to taste
- Pepper to taste

How to prepare:

1. Season pork chops with salt and pepper.
2. Place pork chops in the pot of Ninja Foodi, followed by cabbage, broth, and butter.
3. Close the lid and select "pressure."
4. Set the timer to 12 minutes on "high."
5. Do a natural release and open the lid.
6. Serve and enjoy.

Nutritional Values:

Calories 594 , Total Fat 45.8 g , Saturated Fat 19.1 g , Cholesterol 150 mg , Sodium 463 mg , Total Carbs 7.2 g , Fiber 3 g , Sugar 4.1 g , Protein 37.2 g

BBQ Pork Chops

Preparation time: 10 minutes
Cooking time: 16 minutes
Total time: 26 minutes
Servings: 6

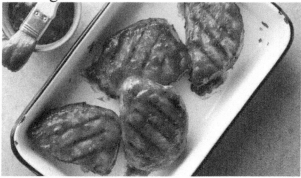

Ingredients:

- 6 lbs pork chops
- ½ cup sugar-free bbq sauce
- Salt to taste
- Pepper to taste

How to prepare:

1. Take a meat tenderizer and tenderize the chops.
2. Season chops with salt and pepper.
3. Take a bowl and add bbq, chops and mix well.
4. Refrigerate chops for 6-8 hours.
5. Arrange chops on "coo and crisp basket" and this basket in the Ninja Foodi.
6. Close the lid and select "air crisp."
7. Set timer for 16 minutes at 355 degrees F.
8. Flip chops halfway through.
9. Press stop, open the lid and serve.

Nutritional Values:

Calories 1472 , Total Fat 112.7 g , Saturated Fat 42.2 g , Cholesterol 390 mg , Sodium 725 mg , Total Carbs 4 g , Fiber 0 g , Sugar 0 g , Protein 101.9 g

Seasoned Pork Tenderloin

Preparation time: 10 minutes
Cooking time: 29 minutes
Total time: 39 minutes
Servings: 3

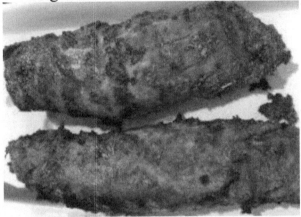

Ingredients:

- 1 lb pork tenderloin
- 2 tablespoons Mrs. Dash seasoning
- 2 cups beef broth
- 2 tablespoons olive oil
- Salt to taste
- Pepper to taste

How to prepare:

1. Season pork with seasoning, salt, and pepper.
2. Turn on the Ninja Foodi and select sauté.
3. All oil and sauté for 3 minutes.
4. Add pork and cook for 2 minutes on each side.
5. Transfer pork in a plate.
6. Pour broth in the pot of Ninja Foodi.
7. Place trivet in the pot and pork on the trivet.
8. Close the lid and select "bake/roast."
9. Set the timer to 25 minutes at 350 degrees and press stop.
10. Open the lid and transfer pork tenderloin on cutting board.
11. Serve and enjoy.

Nutritional Values:

Calories 322 , Total Fat 15.6 g , Saturated Fat 3.4 g , Cholesterol 110 mg , Sodium 645 mg , Total Carbs 0.6 g , Fiber 0 g , Sugar 0.5 g , Protein 42.8 g

Spicy Pork Loin

Preparation time: 10 minutes
Cooking time: 38 minutes
Total time: 48 minutes
Servings: 10

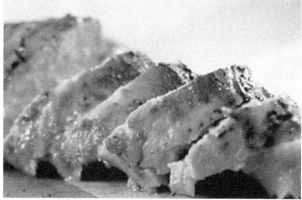

Ingredients:

- 3 lbs pork loin, boneless
- 2 teaspoons smoked paprika
- 1 teaspoon garlic powder
- 2 cups of water
- Olive oil cooking spray
- Salt to taste
- Pepper to taste

How to prepare:

1. Grease the pot of Ninja Foodi and select sauté.
2. Add oil and heat it for 4 minutes.
3. Add pork loin and cook for 3-4 minutes on each side.
4. Transfer pork on a plate.
5. Pour broth in a pot of Ninja Foodi.
6. Place pork on trivet and trivet in the pot.
7. Close the lid and set the valve to seal.
8. Select "pressure" and set the timer for 30 minutes on "high."
9. Do a natural release for 5 minutes and then quick release, open the lid.
10. Transfer pork on a cutting board cut them in slices and serve.

Nutritional Values:

Calories 331 , Total Fat 19 g , Saturated Fat 7.1 g , Cholesterol 109 mg , Sodium 102 mg , Total Carbs 0.4 g , Fiber 0.2 g , Sugar 0.1 g , Protein 37.3 g

Shredded Pork Shoulder

Preparation time: 10 minutes
Cooking time: 38 minutes
Total time: 48 minutes
Servings: 6

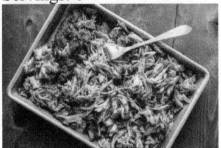

Ingredients:

- 2 lbs pork shoulder, boneless and cubed
- 3 tablespoons lemon juice
- 2 teaspoons lemon zest
- ½ teaspoon red chili powder
- ½ cup chicken broth
- 6 garlic cloves, crushed
- 1 teaspoon dried oregano
- 1 teaspoon ground cumin
- ½ onion, peeled
- 1 tablespoon parsley, chopped
- Salt to taste
- Pepper to taste

How to prepare:

1. Place pork shoulder, lemon juice, lemon zest, chili powder, oregano, cumin, salt, pepper in the pot and stir to combine.
2. Top with onion, broth and close the lid.
3. Select "pressure" and set the timer to 20 minutes at "high."
4. Do a quick release and open the lid.
5. Remove onion and shred the meat.
6. Select sauté and sauté for 10 minutes on "Md:Hi".
7. Close the lid and select "broil."
8. Broil for 8 minutes and open the lid.
9. Serve and enjoy.

Nutritional Values:

Calories 458 , Total Fat 32.7 g , Saturated Fat 12 g , Cholesterol 136 mg , Sodium 199 mg , Total Carbs 2.7 g , Fiber 0.6 g , Sugar 0.7 g , Protein 36.1 g

Graceful Seafood & Fish Recipes

Salmon Stew

Preparation time: 10 minutes
Cooking time: 11 minutes
Total time: 21 minutes
Servings: 3

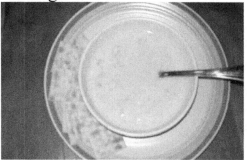

Ingredients:

- 1 cup homemade fish broth
- Salt and black pepper, to taste
- 1 medium onion, chopped
- 1 pound salmon fillet, cubed
- 1 tablespoon butter

How to prepare:

1. Season salmon with salt and pepper.
2. Turn on the Ninja Foodi and select sauté.
3. Add butter, onions and sauté for 3 minutes.
4. Add in salmon and fish broth.
5. Close the lid and select "pressure."
6. Set a timer for 8 minutes and do a natural release.
7. Dish out and serve.

Nutritional Values:

Calories 272 , Total Fat 14.2 g , Saturated Fat 4.1 g , Cholesterol 82 mg , Sodium 275 mg , Total Carbs 4.4 g , Fiber 1.1 g , Sugar 1.9 g , Protein 32.1 g

Paprika Shrimp

Preparation time: 10 minutes
Cooking time: 15 minutes
Total time: 25 minutes
Servings: 3

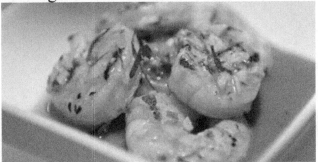

Ingredients:

- 1 teaspoon smoked paprika
- 3 tablespoons butter
- 1 pound tiger shrimps
- Salt, to taste

How to prepare:

1. Take a bowl and add all ingredients in it.
2. Mix well and marinate shrimps in it.
3. Grease pot of Ninja Foodi and add butter in it.
4. Add in seasoned shrimps and press "bake/roast."
5. Set the timer to 15 minutes at 355 degrees F.
6. Serve and enjoy.

Nutritional Values:

Calories 173 , Total Fat 8.3 g , Saturated Fat 1.3 g , Cholesterol 221 mg , Sodium 332 mg , Total Carbs 0.1 g , Fiber 0.1 g , Sugar 0 g , Protein 23.8 g

Butter Fish

Preparation time: 15 minutes
Cooking time: 30 minutes
Total time: 45 minutes
Servings: 3

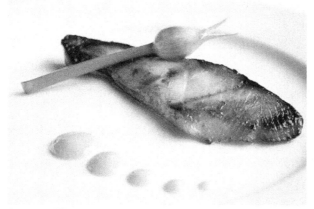

Ingredients:

- 1 pound salmon fillets
- 2 tablespoons ginger-garlic paste
- 3 green chilies, chopped
- Salt and black pepper, to taste
- ¾ cup butter

How to prepare:

1. Season salmon with salt, pepper and ginger garlic paste.
2. Place salmon in Ninja Foodi and top with butter and green chilies.
3. Close the lid.
4. Select "bake/roast" and set the timer for 30 minutes at 360 degrees F.
5. Open the lid, serve and enjoy.

Nutritional Values:

Calories 507 , Total Fat 45.9 g , Saturated Fat 22.9 g , Cholesterol 142 mg , Sodium 296 mg , Total Carbs 2.4 g , Fiber 0.1 g , Sugar 0.2 g , Protein 22.8 g

Delicious Shrimps

Preparation time: 15 minutes
Cooking time: 15 minutes
Total time: 30 minutes
Servings: 3

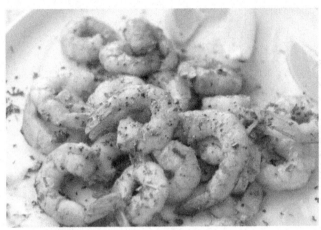

Ingredients:

- 2 tablespoons butter
- ½ teaspoon smoked paprika
- 1 pound shrimps, peeled and deveined
- Lemongrass stalks
- 1 red chili pepper, seeded and chopped

How to prepare:

1. Take a bowl and mix all ingredients in it except lemongrass.
2. Marinate for 1 hour.
3. Add this mixture in ninja pot and close the lid.
4. Select "bake/roast" and set the timer to 15 minutes at 345 degrees F.
5. Open the lid and serve.

Nutritional Values:

Calories 251 , Total Fat 10.3 g , Saturated Fat 5.7 g , Cholesterol 339 mg , Sodium 424 mg , Total Carbs 3 g , Fiber 0.2 g , Sugar 0.1 g , Protein 34.6 g

Sweet and Sour Fish

Preparation time: 15 minutes
Cooking time: 6 minutes
Total time: 21 minutes
Servings: 3

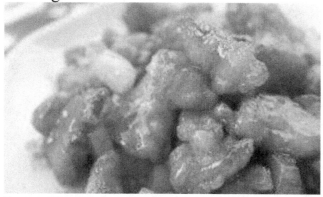

Ingredients:

- 2 drops liquid stevia
- ¼ cup butter
- 1 pound fish chunks
- 1 tablespoon vinegar
- Salt and black pepper, to taste

How to prepare:

1. Turn on the Ninja Foodi and select sauté.
2. Add in butter, fish and sauté for 3 minutes.
3. Add in stevia, salt, pepper and select "air crisp."
4. Cook for 3 minutes at 360 degrees F.
5. Serve and enjoy.

Nutritional Values:

Calories 274 , Total Fat 15.4 g , Saturated Fat 9.7 g , Cholesterol 54 mg , Sodium 604 mg , Total Carbs 2.8 g , Fiber 0 g , Sugar 0 g , Protein 33.2g

Buttery Scallops

Preparation time: 15 minutes
Cooking time: 15 minutes
Total time: 30 minutes
Servings: 6

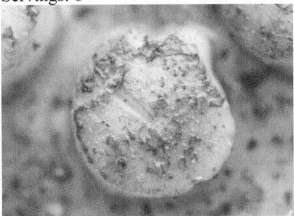

Ingredients:

- 4 garlic cloves, minced
- 4 tablespoons fresh rosemary, chopped
- 2 pounds sea scallops
- ½ cup butter
- Salt and black pepper, to taste

How to prepare:

1. Turn on the Ninja Foodi and select sauté.
2. Add in butter, rosemary, garlic and sauté for 1 minute.
3. Add in scallops, salt, pepper and sauté for 2 minutes.
4. Select "air crisp" for 3 minutes at 350 degrees F.
5. Dish out and serve.

Nutritional Values:

Calories 279 , Total Fat 16.8 g , Saturated Fat 10 g , Cholesterol 91 mg , Sodium 354 mg , Total Carbs 5.7 g , Fiber 1 g , Sugar 0 g , Protein 25.8 g

Buffalo Fish

Preparation time: 15 minutes
Cooking time: 11 minutes
Total time: 26 minutes
Servings: 6

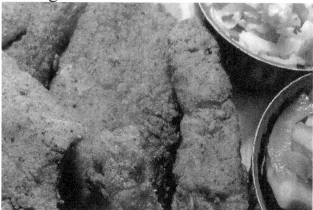

Ingredients:

- 6 tablespoons butter
- ¾ cup Franks red hot sauce
- 6 fish fillets
- Salt and black pepper, to taste
- 2 teaspoons garlic powder

How to prepare:

1. Turn on the Ninja Foodi and select sauté.
2. Add in butter, fish and sauté for 3 minutes.
3. Add in garlic powder, salt, pepper.
4. Select "bake/roast" for 8 minutes at 340 degrees F.
5. Dish out and serve.

Nutritional Values:

Calories 317 , Total Fat 22.7 g , Saturated Fat 9.9 g , Cholesterol 61 mg , Sodium 659 mg , Total Carbs 16.4 g , Fiber 0.6 g , Sugar 0.2 g , Protein 13.6 g

Cod with Herbs

Preparation time: 10 minutes
Cooking time: 8 minutes
Total time: 18 minutes
Servings: 6

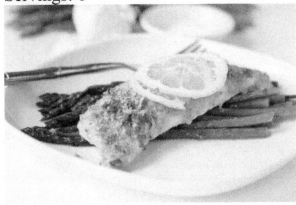

Ingredients:

- 4 garlic cloves, minced
- 2 teaspoons soy sauce
- ¼ cup butter
- 6 eggs
- 2 small onions, chopped finely
- 3 (4-ounce) skinless cod fish fillets, cut into rectangular pieces
- 2 green chilies, chopped finely
- Salt and black pepper, to taste

How to prepare:

1. Take a bowl and add all ingredients in it except cod.
2. Mix well and cover each cod fillet in this mixture and set aside.
3. Place trivet in pot and codon a trivet.
4. Lock the lid and select "air crisp."
5. Set the timer to 8 minutes at 330 degrees F.
6. Open the lid, serve and enjoy.

Nutritional Values:

Calories 409 , Total Fat 25.2 g , Saturated Fat 12.6 g , Cholesterol 430 mg , Sodium 363 mg , Total Carbs 7 g , Fiber 1.1 g , Sugar 3 g , Protein 37.9 g

Glazed Salmon

Preparation time: 10 minutes
Cooking time: 13 minutes
Total time: 23 minutes
Servings: 2

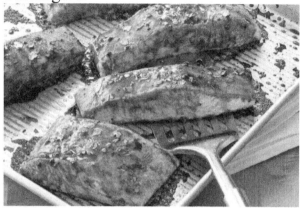

Ingredients:

- 3 tablespoons low sodium soy sauce
- 2 teaspoons lemon juice
- 2 salmon fillets
- 2 teaspoons water

How to prepare:

1. Take a bowl and add all ingredients in it except salmon.
2. Take a small bowl and reserve half of this mixture.
3. Add salmon in remaining mixture and coat it well.
4. Refrigerate salmon for 2 hours.
5. Turn on the Ninja Foodi and place the trivet in it and salmon on the trivet.
6. Close the lid and select "air crisp."
7. Set the timer to 13 minutes at 355 degrees F.
8. Flip halfway through.
9. Open the lid and serve.

Nutritional Values:

Calories 251 , Total Fat 11.1 g , Saturated Fat 1.6 g , Cholesterol 78 mg , Sodium 980 mg , Total Carbs 2.4 g , Fiber 0.2 g , Sugar 0.6 g , Protein 36 g

Cajun Salmon

Preparation time: 15 minutes
Cooking time: 8 minutes
Total time: 23 minutes
Servings: 2

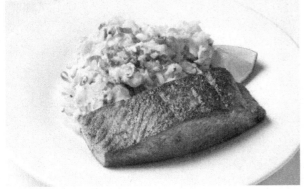

Ingredients:
- 2 tablespoons Cajun seasoning
- 2 salmon fillets

How to prepare:
1. Rub salmon with Cajun seasoning and set it aside.
2. Place salmon on trivet and trivet in the Ninja Foodi.
3. Close the lid and select "air crisp."
4. Select timer to 4 minutes at 390 degrees F.
5. Open the lid and serve.

Nutritional Values:
Calories 235 , Total Fat 11 g , Saturated Fat 1.6 g , Cholesterol 78 mg , Sodium 228 mg , Total Carbs 0 g , Fiber 0 g , Sugar 0 g , Protein 34.7 g

Side Dishes

Sweet Potato Gratin

Preparation time: 10 minutes
Cooking time: 8 minutes
Total time: 18 minutes
Servings: 8

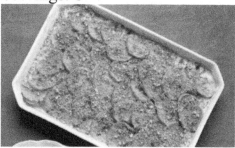

Ingredients:

- 2 tablespoons butter
- 3 tablespoons all-purpose flour
- 2 cups heavy cream, warm
- 2 teaspoons kosher salt
- 1 teaspoon pumpkin pie spice
- ¼ cup of water
- 3 sweet potatoes, peeled and cubed
- 1¼ cups cheddar cheese, shredded
- ½ cup walnuts, chopped

How to prepare:

1. Select sauté on Ninja Foodi.
2. Let it heat for 5 minutes.
3. Add in butter and let it melt.
4. Add in flour and stir together.
5. Cook it for 2 minutes and add in cream. Stir continuously.
6. Add in salt, pumpkin pie spice and mix well to combine.
7. Add in water and let it simmer for 3 minutes.
8. Add in potatoes and close the lid.
9. Select "pressure" and set the timer to 1 minute at "low."
10. Do a quick release.
11. Open the lid, add in shredded cheese and mix well.
12. Top it with remaining nuts and cheese.
13. Close the lid and select "broil" and set the timer to 5 minutes.
14. Open the lid and let cool before serving.

Nutritional Values:

Calories 383 , Total Fat 31.5 g , Saturated Fat 17.2 g , Cholesterol 90 mg , Sodium 881 mg , Total Carbs 13.1 g , Fiber 2.1 g , Sugar 3 g , Protein 13.3 g

Cauliflower Gratin

Preparation time: 10 minutes
Cooking time: 15 minutes
Total time: 25 minutes

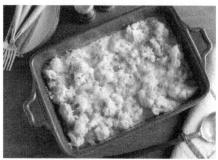

Servings: 4

Ingredients:

- 1 cup beer
- 1 head cauliflower, cut in florets
- 2 teaspoons kosher salt
- 1 pinch nutmeg, ground
- ¼ cup dried raisins
- ½ cup Italian bread crumbs
- ½ cup parmesan, grated
- ½ cup heavy cream
- 1 tablespoon instant flour

How to prepare:

1. Pour beer in the pot of the Ninja Foodi.
2. Add in cauliflower, salt, pepper, currants, and nutmeg.
3. Close the lid and select "pressure."
4. Set the timer to 2 minutes on "high."
5. While the mixture is cooking, take a bowl and stir together crumbs and cheese and set aside.
6. Take another bowl and stir in flour and cream.
7. Do a quick release and open the lid.
8. Add in flour mixture and select sauté.
9. Bring sauce to a boil, add in crumbs mixture.
10. Close the lid and select "air crisp" with a timer 10 minutes at 390 degrees F.
11. Cook until top is golden brown.

Nutritional Values:

Calories 246 , Total Fat 10.6 g , Saturated Fat 6.4 g , Cholesterol 31 mg , Sodium 1671 mg , Total Carbs 25.2 g , Fiber 2.6 g , Sugar 8 g , Protein 10.1 g

Mashed Cheesy Potatoes

Preparation time: 5 minutes
Cooking time: 7 minutes
Total time: 12 minutes
Servings: 4

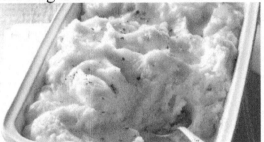

Ingredients:

- 3 russet potatoes, peeled and cut in pieces
- 1 cup of water
- ¼ cup butter, melted
- 1 cup heavy cream
- ½ cup cheddar cheese, shredded
- 1 tablespoon kosher salt
- ½ teaspoon ground black pepper

How to prepare:

1. Add in potatoes and water in the Ninja Foodi pot.
2. Close the lid and select "pressure."
3. Set the timer to 7 minutes at "high."
4. Do a quick release.
5. Open the lid and mash all the ingredients until desired consistency is reached.

Nutritional Values:

Calories 373 , Total Fat 27.5 g , Saturated Fat 17.2 g , Cholesterol 86 mg , Sodium 1936 mg , Total Carbs 26.3 g , Fiber 3.9 g , Sugar 2 g , Protein 7 g

Fried Pickles

Preparation time: 15 minutes
Cooking time: 10 minutes
Total time: 25 minutes
Servings: 6

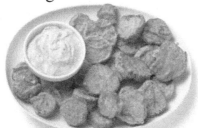

Ingredients:

- 20 dill pickle slices
- ¼ cup all-purpose flour
- 1/8 teaspoon baking powder
- 3 tablespoons beer
- 1/8 teaspoon kosher salt
- 2 tablespoons water
- 2 tablespoons cornstarch
- 1½ cup panko bread crumbs
- 1 teaspoon paprika
- 1 teaspoon garlic powder
- ¼ teaspoon cayenne pepper
- 2 tablespoons canola oil, divided

How to prepare:

1. Dry the pickle slices and place them in the freezer.
2. In a mixing bowl, add flour, baking powder, beer, seltzer water, 2 tablespoons water, salt.
3. Mix until smooth.
4. Take a shallow bowl and place cornstarch in it.
5. Take another bowl and add paprika, crumbs, garlic powder, cayenne pepper in it. Mix well.
6. Coat pickles with cornstarch and then crumbs batter.
7. Place pickles on basket and basket in Ninja Foodi.
8. Select "air fry" with the timer to 3 minutes at 360 degrees F.
9. Serve immediately after frying.

Nutritional Values:

Calories 470 , Total Fat 10.1 g , Saturated Fat 1.6 g , Cholesterol 0 mg , Sodium 1058 mg , Total Carbs 79.1 g , Fiber 5.1 g , Sugar 6.6 g , Protein 14 g

Potato Wedges

Preparation time: 10 minutes
Cooking time: 21 minutes
Total time: 31 minutes
Servings: 4

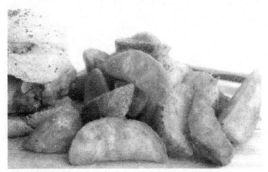

Ingredients:

- ½ cup of water
- 4 potatoes, cut into wedges
- 2 tablespoons extra virgin olive oil, divided
- 1 tablespoon oregano leaves, minced
- 4 cloves garlic, minced
- 1 lemon juice
- 2 tablespoons kosher salt
- 1 teaspoon black pepper

How to prepare:

1. Add in potatoes in the basket in the pot and close the lid.
2. Select "pressure" and set the timer to 3 minutes at "low."
3. While potatoes are cooking, take a small bowl and add olive oil, oregano, garlic, salt, pepper and lemon juice in it. Set it aside.
4. Do a quick release and open the lid.
5. Add remaining olive oil over potatoes.
6. Close lid and select "air crisp" to 18 minutes at 400 degrees F.
7. Open the lid, toss with oregano and serve.

Nutritional Values:

Calories 217 , Total Fat 7.4 g , Saturated Fat 1.1 g , Cholesterol 0 mg , Sodium 3503 mg , Total Carbs 35.6 g , Fiber 5.8 g , Sugar 2.6 g , Protein 4 g

Baked Apples

Preparation time: 10 minutes
Cooking time: 45 minutes
Total time: 55 minutes
Servings: 4

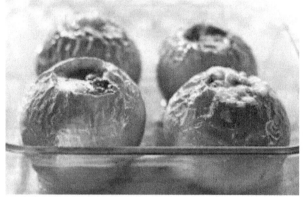

Ingredients:

- 2 apples, cut in half and cored
- 1 lemon juice
- 4 teaspoons light brown sugar
- ¼ cup butter, cut in 16 pieces
- 8 teaspoons granulated sugar

How to prepare:

1. Pierce each apple with a fork around 6 times.
2. Insert crisper plate in basket and basket in Ninja Foodi.
3. Select "air fry" for 3 minutes at 325 degrees F.
4. Place aluminum foil on basket and apples on it.
5. Sprinkle with brown sugar, lemon juice and top each apple with butter.
6. Select "air fry" with timer 45 minutes at 325 degrees F.
7. Halfway through select pause and sprinkle granulated on top and then select start.
8. Serve and enjoy.

Nutritional Values:

Calories 204 , Total Fat 11.8 g , Saturated Fat 7.4 g , Cholesterol 31 mg , Sodium 86 mg , Total Carbs 26.6 g , Fiber 2.8 g , Sugar 22.8 g , Protein 0.5 g

Sweet Potato Tots

Preparation time: 15 minutes
Cooking time: 23 minutes
Total time: 38 minutes
Servings: 6

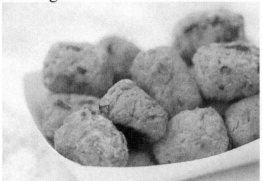

Ingredients:

- 3 sweet potatoes, peeled and cubed
- 4 sprigs fresh thyme
- ¼ teaspoon cinnamon
- 1½ tablespoons kosher salt, divided
- 1½ cups water
- ½ cup cornstarch, divided
- 4 cups panko bread crumbs
- 2 teaspoons ground cumin
- 1 teaspoon chili powder
- 1 teaspoon black pepper

How to prepare:

1. Add sweet potatoes, thyme, cinnamon, 1 teaspoon kosher salt in the pot.
2. Close the lid and select "pressure."
3. Set the timer to 8 minutes at "high."
4. Do a quick release.
5. Open the lid and strain potatoes in a colander.
6. Place basket in the pot.
7. Mash potatoes and add 2 tablespoons cornstarch and mix until smooth.
8. Take a bowl and add remaining salt, cornstarch, cumin, crumbs, pepper, and chili powder.
9. Make round balls of potato mixture.
10. Coat them with crumbs mixture and place in freezer for an hour.
11. Close lid of the pot, then select "air crisp" for 5 minutes at 400 degrees F.
12. Now the pot is preheated, spray cooking oil in the basket and add tots in it.
13. Select "air crisp" for 15 minutes at 400 degrees F.

14. Dish out and serve.

Nutritional Values:

Calories 374 , Total Fat 4.1 g , Saturated Fat 0.9 g , Cholesterol 0 mg , Sodium 6938 mg , Total Carbs 72.7 g , Fiber 4.8 g , Sugar 4.9 g , Protein 10.8 g

Thai Chili Chicken Wings

Preparation time: 15 minutes
Cooking time: 20 minutes
Total time: 35 minutes
Servings: 6

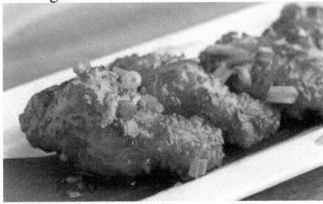

Ingredients:

- ½ cup of water
- 2 lbs frozen chicken wings
- 2 tablespoons canola oil
- 2 tablespoons Thai chili sauce
- 2 teaspoons kosher salt
- 2 teaspoons sesame seeds, for garnish

How to prepare:

1. Pour water in pot and place wings into the pot.
2. Close the lid and select "pressure."
3. Set the timer to 12 minutes at "high."
4. Do a quick release and open the lid.
5. Toss wings with oil and close the lid.
6. Select "air crisp" to 15 minutes at 390 degrees F.
7. After 7 minutes open lid, toss wings and resume the process.
8. Take a bowl and add the chili sauce, salt and mix well.
9. Open the lid and place wings in the sauce and serve.

Nutritional Values:

Calories 127 , Total Fat 10.5 g , Saturated Fat 1.9 g , Cholesterol 25 mg , Sodium 1119 mg , Total Carbs 1.9 g , Fiber 0.1 g , Sugar 1.3 g , Protein 6.2 g

Fish n Chips

Preparation time: 10 minutes
Cooking time: 10 minutes
Total time: 20 minutes
Servings: 4

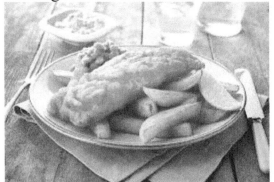

Ingredients:

- 1 cup of rice flour
- 1 teaspoon kosher salt
- 2 eggs, beaten
- 7.35 ounces salt & vinegar, crushed
- 5 frozen flounder fillets, cut in half

How to prepare:

1. Take a bowl and add flour, salt and mix well.
2. Add eggs to another bowl.
3. Take the 3rd bowl and place crushed chips.
4. Coat fillets with flour, then eggs, then chips mixture.
5. Set it aside and freeze for 2 hours.
6. Place fillets on basket and basket in Ninja Foodi.
7. Select "air crisp" for 10 minutes at 390 degrees F.
8. Dish out and serve.

Nutritional Values:

Calories 579 , Total Fat 20.9 g , Saturated Fat 4.9 g , Cholesterol 150 mg , Sodium 1223 mg , Total Carbs 57.6 g , Fiber 2.8 g , Sugar 1.9 g , Protein 35 g

Chicken Tacos

Preparation time: 10 minutes
Cooking time: 35 minutes
Total time: 45 minutes
Servings: 12

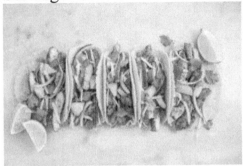

Ingredients:

- 4 cloves garlic, peeled
- 1 can chipotle peppers in adobo sauce
- 1 small onion, peeled and cut in quarters
- 1 can diced tomatoes
- 2 lbs chicken breasts, uncooked and skinless
- 1 cup chicken stock
- 1 tablespoon kosher salt
- 1 teaspoon black pepper
- ¼ cup parsley, chopped and fresh
- 12 corn or flour tortillas, 6 inches

How to prepare:

1. Take a blender and add garlic, adobo sauce, onion, tomatoes and blend till smooth.
2. Add in chicken stock, vegetables, salt, pepper in the pot and mix well.
3. Close the lid and select "pressure."
4. Set the timer to 25 minutes on "high."
5. Do a quick release and open the lid.
6. Select sauté and let liquid simmer for 10 minutes.
7. Shred chicken and assemble tacos in tortillas and serve.

Nutritional Values:

Calories 208 , Total Fat 6.5 g , Saturated Fat 1.7 g , Cholesterol 68 mg , Sodium 751 mg , Total Carbs 13.1 g , Fiber 2.3 g , Sugar 1.3 g , Protein 23.8 g

Tasty Dessert Recipes

Peanut Butter Cups

Preparation time: 15 minutes
Cooking time: 30 minutes
Total time: 45 minutes
Servings: 3

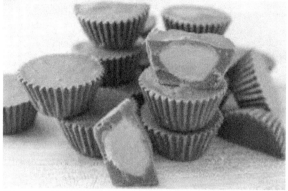

Ingredients:

- 1 cup butter
- ¼ cup heavy cream
- 2 ounces unsweetened chocolate
- ¼ cup peanut butter, separated
- 4 packets stevia

How to prepare:

1. Melt the peanut butter and butter in a bowl and stir well with unsweetened chocolate, stevia, and cream.
2. Mix well and pour the mixture in a baking mold.
3. Put the baking mold in the Ninja Foodi and press "Bake/Roast."
4. Set the timer for 30 minutes at 360 degrees F and dish out to serve.

Nutritional Values:

Calories 479 , Total Fat 51.5 g , Saturated Fat 29.7 g , Cholesterol 106 mg , Sodium 69 mg , Total Carbs 7.7 g , Fiber 2.7 g , Sugar 1.4 g , Protein 5.2 g

Crème Brulee

Serve and enjoy.
Preparation time: 15 minutes
Cooking time: 15 minutes
Total time: 30 minutes
Servings: 4

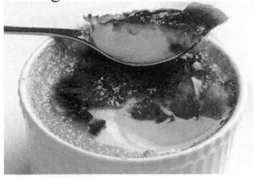

Ingredients:

- 1 cup heavy cream
- ½ tablespoon vanilla extract
- 3 egg yolks
- 1 pinch salt
- ¼ cup stevia

How to prepare:

1. Take a bowl and mix egg yolks, vanilla extract, heavy cream, and salt.
2. Divide the mixture into ramekins evenly and transfer them on the basket of Ninja Foodi.
3. Press "Bake/Roast" and set the timer for 15 minutes at 365 degrees F.
4. Take out and cover the ramekins with a plastic wrap.
5. Refrigerate for 3 hours.

Nutritional Values:

Calories 149 , Total Fat 14.5 g , Saturated Fat 8.1 g , Cholesterol 56 mg , Sodium 56 mg , Total Carbs 1.6 g , Fiber 0 g , Sugar 0.3 g , Protein 2.6 g

Chocolate Brownies

Preparation time: 15 minutes
Cooking time: 32 minutes
Total time: 47 minutes
Servings: 4

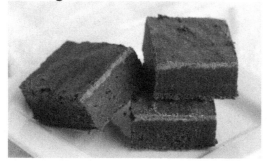

Ingredients:

- 3 eggs
- ½ cup butter
- ½ cup sugar-free chocolate chips
- 2 scoops stevia
- 1 teaspoon vanilla extract

How to prepare:

1. Take a bowl and mix eggs, stevia, and vanilla extract.
2. Pour this mixture in the blender and blend until smooth.
3. Put the butter and chocolate in the pot of Ninja Foodi and press sauté.
4. Sauté for 2 minutes until the chocolate is melted.
5. Add the melted chocolate into egg mixture.
6. Pour the mixture in the baking mold and place it in the Ninja Foodi.
7. Press "Bake/Roast" and set the timer for about 30 minutes at 360 degrees F.
8. Bake for about 30 minutes, cut into pieces and serve.

Nutritional Values:

Calories 266 , Total Fat 26.9 g , Saturated Fat 15.8 g , Cholesterol 184 mg , Sodium 218 mg , Total Carbs 2.5 g , Fiber 0 g , Sugar 0.4 g , Protein 4.5 g

Cream Crepes

Preparation time: 15 minutes
Cooking time: 16 minutes
Total time: 31 minutes
Servings: 6

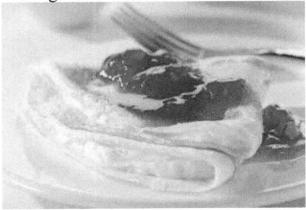

Ingredients:

- 1½ teaspoons Splenda
- 3 organic eggs
- 3 tablespoons coconut flour
- ½ cup heavy cream
- 3 tablespoons coconut oil, melted and divided

How to prepare:

1. Take a bowl and mix 1½ tablespoons of coconut oil, Splenda, eggs, and salt.
2. Add the coconut flour and continuously stir.
3. Add in the heavy cream and stir continuously until smooth.
4. Press sauté on Ninja Foodi and pour about ¼ of the mixture in the pot.
5. Sauté for 2 minutes on each side and dish out.
6. Repeat until mixture ends and serve.

Nutritional Values:

Calories 145 , Total Fat 13.1 g , Saturated Fat 9.1 g , Cholesterol 96 mg , Sodium 35 mg , Total Carbs 4 g , Fiber 1.5 g , Sugar 1.2 g , Protein 3.5 g

Nut Porridge

Preparation time: 15 minutes
Cooking time: 10 minutes
Total time: 25 minutes
Servings: 4

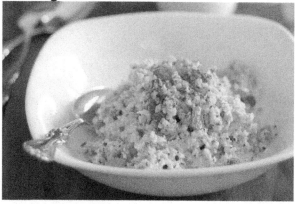

Ingredients:

- 4 teaspoons coconut oil, melted
- 1 cup pecans, halved
- 2 cups of water
- 2 tablespoons stevia
- 1 cup cashew nuts, raw and unsalted

How to prepare:

1. Put the cashew nuts and pecans in the precision processor and pulse till they are in chunks.
2. Put this mixture into the pot of Ninja Foodi and stir in water, coconut oil and stevia.
3. Select sauté on Ninja Foodi and cook for 15 minutes.
4. Serve and enjoy.

Nutritional Values:

Calories 260 , Total Fat 22.9 g , Saturated Fat 7.3 g , Cholesterol 0 mg , Sodium 9 mg , Total Carbs 12.7 g , Fiber 1.4 g , Sugar 1.8 g , Protein 5.6 g

Lemon Mousse

Preparation time: 15 minutes
Cooking time: 12 minutes
Total time: 27 minutes
Servings: 2

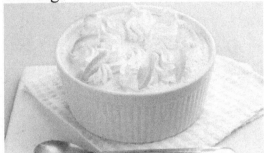

Ingredients:

- 4-ounce cream cheese softened
- ½ cup heavy cream
- 1/8 cup fresh lemon juice
- ½ teaspoon lemon liquid stevia
- 2 pinches salt

How to prepare:

1. Take a bowl and mix cream cheese, heavy cream, lemon juice, salt, and stevia.
2. Pour this mixture into the ramekins and transfer the ramekins in the pot of Ninja Foodi.
3. Select "Bake/Roast" and bake for 12 minutes at 350 degrees F.
4. Pour into the serving glasses and refrigerate for at least 3 hours.
5. Serve and enjoy.

Nutritional Values:

Calories 305 , Total Fat 31 g , Saturated Fat 19.5 g , Cholesterol 103 mg , Sodium 299 mg , Total Carbs 2.7 g , Fiber 0.1 g , Sugar 0.5 g , Protein 5 g

Chocolate Cheesecake

Preparation time: 15 minutes
Cooking time: 15 minutes
Total time: 30 minutes
Servings: 6

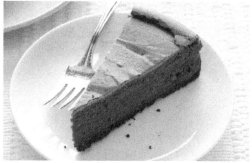

Ingredients:

- 2 cups cream cheese, softened
- 2 eggs
- 2 tablespoons cocoa powder
- 1 teaspoon pure vanilla extract
- ½ cup Swerve

How to prepare:

1. Add in eggs, cocoa powder, vanilla extract, swerve, cream cheese in an immersion blender and blend until smooth.
2. Pour the mixture evenly into mason jars.
3. Put the mason jars in the insert of Ninja Foodi and close the lid.
4. Select "Bake/Roast" and bake for 15 minutes at 360 degrees F.
5. Refrigerate for at least 2 hours.
6. Serve and enjoy.

Nutritional Values:

Calories 244 , Total Fat 24.8 g , Saturated Fat 15.6 g , Cholesterol 32 mg , Sodium 204 mg , Total Carbs 2.1 g , Fiber 0.1 g , Sugar 0.4 g , Protein 4 g

Vanilla Yogurt

Preparation time: 15 minutes
Cooking time: 3 hours
Total time: 3 hours 15 minutes
Servings: 2

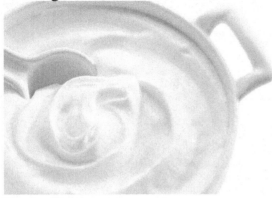

Ingredients:

- ½ cup full-fat milk
- ¼ cup yogurt starter
- 1 cup heavy cream
- ½ tablespoon pure vanilla extract
- 2 scoops stevia

How to prepare:

1. Add in milk, heavy cream, vanilla extract, and stevia in Ninja Foodi.
2. Let yogurt sit and press "slow cooker" and set the timer to 4 hours on "low."
3. Add yogurt starter in 1 cup of milk.
4. Return this mixture to the pot.
5. Close the lid and wrap the Ninja Foodi in small towels.
6. Let yogurt sit for about 9 hours.
7. Dish out, refrigerate and then serve.

Nutritional Values:

Calories 292 , Total Fat 26.2 g , Saturated Fat 16.3 g , Cholesterol 100 mg , Sodium 86 mg , Total Carbs 8.2 g , Fiber 0 g , Sugar 6.6 g , Protein 5.2 g

Coffee Custard

Preparation time: 15 minutes
Cooking time: 10 minutes
Total time: 25 minutes
Servings: 4

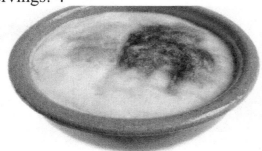

Ingredients:

- 4-ounces mascarpone cream cheese
- 1 teaspoon espresso powder
- ¼ cup unsalted butter
- 4 large organic eggs, whites and yolks separated
- 1 tablespoon water
- ¼ teaspoon cream of tartar
- ½ teaspoon liquid stevia
- ¼ teaspoon monk fruit extract drops

How to prepare:

1. Select sauté and "Lo: Md" on Ninja Foodi and add in butter and cream cheese.
2. Sauté for 3 minutes and mix in espresso powder, egg yolks, and water.
3. Select "low" and cook for 4 minutes.
4. Take a bowl and whisk together egg whites, fruit drops, stevia, cream of tartar.
5. Pour in the egg white mixture in the mixture present in Ninja Foodi and cook for 3 minutes.
6. Pour it into serving glasses and refrigerate it for 3 hours.
7. Serve and enjoy.

Nutritional Values:

Calories 292 , Total Fat 26.2 g , Saturated Fat 16.3 g , Cholesterol 100 mg , Sodium 86 mg , Total Carbs 8.2 g , Fiber 0 g , Sugar 6.6 g , Protein 5.2 g

Chocolate Fudge

Preparation time: 15 minutes
Cooking time: 6 hours
Total time: 6 hours 15 minutes
Servings: 24

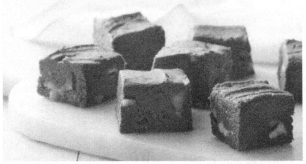

Ingredients:

- ½ teaspoon organic vanilla extract
- 1 cup heavy whipping cream
- 2-ounce butter softened
- 2-ounce 70% dark chocolate, finely chopped

How to prepare:

1. Select sauté and "Md: Hi" on Ninja Foodi and add in vanilla and heavy cream.
2. Sauté for 5 minutes at "low."
3. Sauté for 10 minutes and add in butter and chocolate.
4. Sauté for 2 minutes and pour this mixture in a serving dish.
5. Refrigerate it for some hours and serve.

Nutritional Values:

Calories 292 , Total Fat 26.2 g , Saturated Fat 16.3 g , Cholesterol 100 mg , Sodium 86 mg , Total Carbs 8.2 g , Fiber 0 g , Sugar 6.6 g , Protein 5.2 g

Nice Snack Recipes

Stuffed Eggs

Preparation time: 5 minutes
Cooking time: 5 minutes
Total time: 10 minutes
Servings: 6

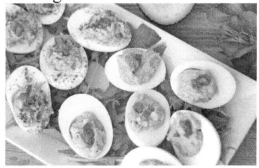

Ingredients:

- ½ tablespoon fresh lemon juice
- 1 medium ripe avocado, peeled, pitted and chopped
- 6 organic eggs, boiled, peeled and cut in half lengthwise
- Salt, to taste
- ½ cup fresh watercress, trimmed

How to prepare:

1. Place trivet at the bottom of Ninja Foodi and add water.
2. Place watercress on the basket and close the lid.
3. Select "pressure" and set the timer to 3 minutes.
4. Do a quick release.
5. Drain the watercress completely.
6. Take a bowl and add all egg yolks in it.
7. Add in watercress, avocado, lemon juice, and salt and mash with a fork thoroughly.
8. Place mixture in egg whites and serve.

Nutritional Values:

Calories 132 , Total Fat 10.9 g , Saturated Fat 2.7 g , Cholesterol 164 mg , Sodium 65 mg , Total Carbs 3.3 g , Fiber 2.3 g , Sugar 0.5 g , Protein 6.3 g

Cheese Casserole

Preparation time: 10 minutes
Cooking time: 22 minutes
Total time: 32 minutes
Servings: 6

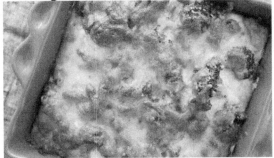

Ingredients:

- 16-ounce marinara sauce
- 10-ounce parmesan, shredded
- 2 tablespoons olive oil
- 16-ounce mozzarella cheese, shredded
- 2 pounds sausages, scrambled

How to prepare:

1. Grease the pot of Ninja Foodi with add half of the scrambled sausages at the bottom.
2. Layer with half of the marinara sauce and then by half of the mozzarella and Parmesan cheese.
3. Repeat this process once more.
4. Select "bake/roast" and set the timer to 20 minutes at 360 degrees F.
5. Dish out to serve.

Nutritional Values:

Calories 521 , Total Fat 38.8 g , Saturated Fat 12.8 g , Cholesterol 136 mg , Sodium 201 mg , Total Carbs 6 g , Fiber 0 g , Sugar 5.4 g , Protein 35.4 g

Avocado Chips

Preparation time: 15 minutes
Cooking time: 10 minutes
Total time: 25 minutes
Servings: 4

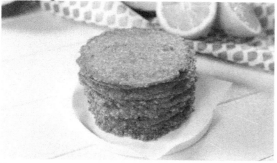

Ingredients:

- 4 tablespoons butter
- 4 raw avocados, peeled and sliced in chips form
- Salt and black pepper, to taste

How to prepare:

1. Season avocado slices with salt and pepper.
2. Grease the pot of Ninja Foodi with butter and add in avocado.
3. Select "air crisp" and set the timer to 10 minutes at 350 degrees F.
4. Dish out and serve.

Nutritional Values:

Calories 391 , Total Fat 38.2 g , Saturated Fat 11 g , Cholesterol 31 mg , Sodium 96 mg , Total Carbs 15 g , Fiber 0.5 g , Sugar 11.8 g , Protein 3.5 g

Scallion Cake

Preparation time: 15 minutes
Cooking time: 20 minutes
Total time: 35 minutes
Servings: 4

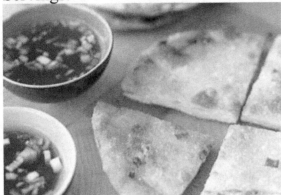

Ingredients:

- ½ cup Parmesan cheese, finely grated
- ½ cup low-fat cottage cheese
- ¼ cup flax seeds meal
- ½ teaspoon baking powder
- 1/3 cup scallion, thinly sliced
- ¼ cup nutritional yeast flakes
- ½ cup raw hemp seeds
- Salt, to taste
- ½ cup almond meal
- 6 organic eggs, beaten

How to prepare:

1. Take a bowl and mix eggs, cottage cheese and set aside.
2. Take another bowl and mix baking powder, hemp seeds, flax seeds meal, almond meal, and salt.
3. Combine the two mixtures and add in scallions.
4. Pour mixture evenly into ramekins and place in the pot of Ninja Foodi.
5. Select "bake/roast" and set the timer to 20 minutes at 345 degrees F.
6. Dish out and serve.

Nutritional Values:

Calories 306 , Total Fat 19.7 g , Saturated Fat 4.7 g , Cholesterol 0 mg , Sodium 398 mg , Total Carbs 10.7 g , Fiber 4.2 g , Sugar 1.3 g , Protein 23.5 g

Mixed Nuts

Preparation time: 10 minutes
Cooking time: 15 minutes
Total time: 25 minutes
Servings: 5

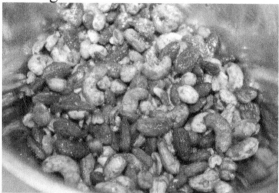

Ingredients:

- 1 tablespoon butter, melted
- ½ cup raw cashew nuts
- 1 cup of raw almonds
- 1 cup of raw peanuts
- Salt, to taste

How to prepare:

1. Place the nuts in the pot of Ninja Foodi and close the lid.
2. Press "air crisp" and set the timer to 10 minutes at 350 degrees F.
3. Remove nuts into a bowl, add in melted butter and salt.
4. Toss well and return the nut mixture into the pot.
5. Select "bake/roast" and bake for 5 minutes.
6. Dish out to serve.

Nutritional Values:

Calories 189 , Total Fat 16.5 g , Saturated Fat 2.2 g , Cholesterol 0 mg , Sodium 19 mg , Total Carbs 6.6 g , Fiber 2.6 g , Sugar 1.3 g , Protein 6.8 g

Asparagus Bites

Preparation time: 10 minutes
Cooking time: 10 minutes
Total time: 20 minutes
Servings: 3

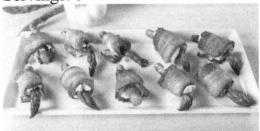

Ingredients:

- 1 cup asparagus
- ½ cup desiccated coconut
- ½ cup feta cheese

How to prepare:

1. Take a dish and place coconut in it, coat asparagus with coconut.
2. Place this asparagus in the pot of Ninja Foodi and top it with feta cheese.
3. Select "air crisp" and set the timer to 10 minutes at 360 degrees F.
4. Dish out and serve.

Nutritional Values:

Calories 135 , Total Fat 10.3 g , Saturated Fat 7.7 g , Cholesterol 33 mg , Sodium 421 mg , Total Carbs 5 g , Fiber 2 g , Sugar 3.1 g , Protein 7 g

Broccoli Bites

Preparation time: 30 minutes
Cooking time: 12 minutes
Total time: 42 minutes
Servings: 6

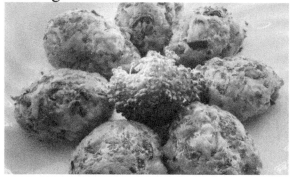

Ingredients:

- 1/3 cup Parmesan cheese, grated
- 2 cups cheddar cheese, grated
- Salt and black pepper, to taste
- 3 eggs, beaten
- 3 cups broccoli florets
- 1 tablespoon olive oil

How to prepare:

1. Put broccoli in a food processor and pulse until crumbled finely.
2. Take a bowl and add in broccoli with the remaining ingredients and mix well.
3. Make small balls from the mixture and refrigerate for 30 minutes.
4. Place balls in the pot of Ninja Foodi and close the lid.
5. Select "air crisp" and set the timer to 12 minutes at 350 degrees F.
6. Open the lid, dish out and serve.

Nutritional Values:

Calories 162 , Total Fat 12.4 g , Saturated Fat 7.6 g , Cholesterol 69 mg , Sodium 263 mg , Total Carbs 1.9 g , Fiber 0.5 g , Sugar 0.5 g , Protein 11.2 g

Zucchini Fries

Preparation time: 15 minutes
Cooking time: 10 minutes
Total time: 25 minutes
Servings: 4

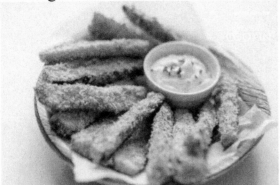

Ingredients:

- 1 pound zucchini, sliced into 2 ½-inch sticks
- Salt, to taste
- 1 cup cream cheese
- 2 tablespoons olive oil

How to prepare:

1. Place zucchini in a colander.
2. Add in salt and cream cheese.
3. Pour oil and zucchini in the pot of Ninja Foodi and close the lid.
4. Select "air crisp" and set the timer to 10 minutes at 365 degrees F.
5. Open the lid, serve and have fun!

Nutritional Values:

Calories 374 , Total Fat 36.6 g , Saturated Fat 18.4 g , Cholesterol 85 mg , Sodium 294 mg , Total Carbs 7.1 g , Fiber 1.7 g , Sugar 2.8 g , Protein 7.7 g

Apple Crisp

Preparation time: 10 minutes
Cooking time: 20 minutes
Total time: 30 minutes
Servings: 5

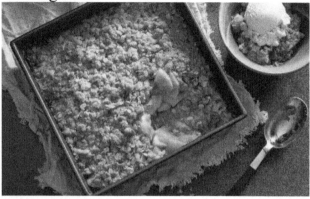

Ingredients:

- 5 apples, cut and peeled into chunks
- 2 teaspoons cinnamon
- 1 teaspoon maple syrup
- ½ teaspoon nutmeg
- ½ cup of water
- 4 tablespoons butter, melted
- ¼ cup brown sugar
- ¼ cup flour
- ¾ cup rolled oats
- ½ teaspoon salt

How to prepare:

1. Spray cooking oil at the bottom of Ninja Foodi.
2. Add all ingredients in it and mix well.
3. Close the lid and select "bake/roast."
4. Set the timer to 14 minutes at "high."
5. Open the lid, dish out and serve.

Nutritional Values:

Calories 301 , Total Fat 10.6 g , Saturated Fat 6.1 g , Cholesterol 24 mg , Sodium 304 mg , Total Carbs 52.7 g , Fiber 7.4 g , Sugar 31.3 g , Protein 3 g

Mixed Veggies

Preparation time: 10 minutes
Cooking time: 12 minutes
Total time: 22 minutes
Servings: 4

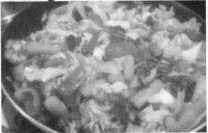

Ingredients:
For vegetables
- 3 tablespoons olive oil
- 1 pound eggplant, cut into 1-inch pieces
- 1 red bell pepper, seeded and chopped
- 1 (3½-ounce) package shiitake mushrooms, sliced
- 2 garlic cloves, chopped
- 1 tablespoon fresh ginger, chopped
- 1 fresh scallion, chopped

For Sauce
- 2 tablespoons low-sodium soy sauce
- 1 tablespoon fresh lemon juice
- 1 teaspoon Erythritol
- ¼ teaspoon red pepper flakes
- Salt and ground black pepper, to taste

How to prepare:
1. Select sauté on Ninja Foodi.
2. Add in oil and let it heat for 3 minutes.
3. Add in vegetables and sauté for 5 minutes.
4. Add in garlic, ginger and sauté for 2 minutes.
5. Take a bowl for sauce and add all sauce ingredients in it. Mix well.
6. Close the lid and select "broil."
7. Set timer to 8 minutes.
8. Open the lid serve and pour sauce over it.

Nutritional Values:
Calories 199 , Total Fat 11.2 g , Saturated Fat 1.6 g , Cholesterol 0 mg , Sodium 748 mg , Total Carbs 27.7 g , Fiber 7.1 g , Sugar 10.9 g , Protein 4 g

Conclusion

Ninja Foodi can serve as a multi-purpose device. No other device can replace it. It is a durable appliance. All of its components are solidly made and assembled so this appliance would last for years in your house. We should surely buy it because it is all in one gadget. It works exceptionally well. Most of the food is cooked well in time because it cooks faster than other appliances. It does an excellent job of pressure cooking and air frying. It's not a good option if you have a small kitchen but, if you can accommodate it, your life will become easier.

Made in the USA
Columbia, SC
15 November 2019

83151496R00072